Geriatric Medicine

Editors

SUSAN E. MEREL
JEFFREY WALLACE

MEDICAL CLINICS
OF NORTH AMERICA

www.medical.theclinics.com

Consulting Editors
DOUGLAS S. PAAUW
EDWARD R. BOLLARD

March 2015 • Volume 99 • Number 2

ELSEVIER

1600 John F. Kennedy Boulevard • Suite 1800 • Philadelphia, Pennsylvania, 19103-2899

http://www.theclinics.com

MEDICAL CLINICS OF NORTH AMERICA Volume 99, Number 2
March 2015 ISSN 0025-7125, ISBN-13: 978-0-323-35659-6

Editor: Jessica McCool
Developmental Editor: Susan Showalter

Medical Clinics of North America (ISSN 0025-7125) is published bimonthly by Elsevier Inc., 360 Park Avenue South, New York, NY 10010-1710. Months of publication are January, March, May, July, September, and November. Business and editorial offices: 1600 John F. Kennedy Boulevard, Suite 1800, Philadelphia, PA 19103-2899. Periodicals postage paid at New York, NY, and additional mailing offices. Subscription prices are USD $255.00 per year (US individuals), $471.00 per year (US institutions), $125.00 per year (US Students), $320.00 per year (Canadian individuals), $612.00 per year (Canadian institutions), $200.00 per year (Canadian and foreign students), $390.00 per year (foreign individuals), and $612.00 per year (foreign institutions). To receive student/resident rate, orders must be accompanied by name of affiliated institution, date of term, and the signature of program/residency coordinator on institution letterhead. Orders will be billed at individual rate until proof of status is received. Foreign air speed delivery is included in all Clinics' subscription prices. All prices are subject to change without notice. **POSTMASTER:** Send address changes to *Medical Clinics of North America*, Elsevier Health Sciences Division, Subscription Customer Service, 3251 Riverport Lane, Maryland Heights, MO 63043. **Customer Service: Telephone: 1-800-654-2452** (U.S. and Canada); **1-314-447-8871** (outside U.S. and Canada). **Fax: 314-447-8029. E-mail: journalscustomerserviceusa@elsevier.com** (for print support); **journalsonlinesupport-usa@elsevier.com** (for online support).

Reprints. For copies of 100 or more of articles in this publication, please contact the Commercial Reprints Department, Elsevier Inc., 360 Park Avenue South, New York, NY 10010-1710. Tel.: 212-633-3874; Fax: 212-633-3820; E-mail: reprints@elsevier.com.

Medical Clinics of North America is also published in Spanish by McGraw-Hill Interamericana Editores S. A., P.O. Box 5-237, 06500 Mexico, D.F., Mexico.

Medical Clinics of North America is covered in *MEDLINE/PubMed (Index Medicus), Current Contents, ASCA, Excerpta Medica, Science Citation Index, and ISI/BIOMED.*

Printed in the United States of America.

PROGRAM OBJECTIVE
The goal of the *Medical Clinics of North America* is to keep practicing physicians up to date with current clinical practice by providing timely articles reviewing the state of the art in patient care.

TARGET AUDIENCE
All practicing physicians and other healthcare professionals.

LEARNING OBJECTIVES
Upon completion of this activity, participants will be able to:
1. Review the management of conditions that effect the elderly population including cognitive complaints, fall risks, diabetes, urinary incontinence, sleep problems, management of pain, and cancer.
2. Discuss appropriate prescribing and important drug interactions in older adults.
3. Describe the management of the geriatric patient with atrial fibrillation and the geriatric patient with hypertension.

ACCREDITATION
The Elsevier Office of Continuing Medical Education (EOCME) is accredited by the Accreditation Council for Continuing Medical Education (ACCME) to provide continuing medical education for physicians.

The EOCME designates this enduring material for a maximum of 15 *AMA PRA Category 1 Credit*(s)™. Physicians should claim only the credit commensurate with the extent of their participation in the activity.

All other health care professionals requesting continuing education credit for this enduring material will be issued a certificate of participation.

DISCLOSURE OF CONFLICTS OF INTEREST
The EOCME assesses conflict of interest with its instructors, faculty, planners, and other individuals who are in a position to control the content of CME activities. All relevant conflicts of interest that are identified are thoroughly vetted by EOCME for fair balance, scientific objectivity, and patient care recommendations. EOCME is committed to providing its learners with CME activities that promote improvements or quality in healthcare and not a specific proprietary business or a commercial interest.

The planning committee, staff, authors and editors listed below have identified no financial relationships or relationships to products or devices they or their spouse/life partner have with commercial interest related to the content of this CME activity:
Kirk M. Anderson, MD; Nidhi Bansal, MBBS; David B. Bekelman, MD, MPH; Edward R. Bollard, MD, DDS; Charlotte Carlson, MD, MPH; Skotti Church, MD; Karlotta Davis, MD, MPH; Ruban Dhaliwal, MD; Joseph M. Dzierzewski, PhD; Karli Edholm, MD, FACP; Brian J. Flynn, MD; Anjali Fortna; Kerry L. Hildreth, MD; Brynne Hunter; Philip A. Kithas, MD, PhD; Sandy Lavery; Hillary D. Lum, MD, PhD; Monica Malec, MD; Jessica McCool; Susan E. Merel, MD; Douglas S. Paauw, MD, MACP; Santha Priya; Nathan Ragle, MD; Juan Carlos Rodriguez, MD; Matthew T. Rondina, MD, MS; Joseph W. Shega, MD; Michael C. Soung, MD, FACP; Judy A. Stevens, PhD; Rebecca L. Sudore, MD; Megan Suermann; Mark A. Supiano, MD; Jan C. Voit, PT; Jeffrey Wallace, MD, MPH; Michi Yukawa, MD, MPH.

The planning committee, staff, authors and editors listed below have identified financial relationships or relationships to products or devices they or their spouse/life partner have with commercial interest related to the content of this CME activity:
Cathy A. Alessi, MD is a consultant/advisor for OptumRX, Inc.
Jane E. Mahoney, MD has royalties/patents with Stepping On Leader's Manual
Elizabeth A. Phelan, MD, MS is a consultant/advisor for Centers for Disease Control and Prevention
Ruth S. Weinstock, MD, PhD has research grants from Biodel Inc., Calibra Medical, Intarcia Therapeutics, Inc., Medtronic, Milan Medical a service of da Vinci Network Services, Novo Nordisk A/S and sanofi-aventis U.S. LLC

UNAPPROVED/OFF-LABEL USE DISCLOSURE
The EOCME requires CME faculty to disclose to the participants:
1. When products or procedures being discussed are off-label, unlabelled, experimental, and/or investigational (not US Food and Drug Administration [FDA] approved); and
2. Any limitations on the information presented, such as data that are preliminary or that represent ongoing research, interim analyses, and/or unsupported opinions. Faculty may discuss information about pharmaceutical agents that is outside of FDA-approved labelling. This information is intended solely for CME and is not intended to promote off-label use of these medications. If you have any

questions, contact the medical affairs department of the manufacturer for the most recent prescribing information.

TO ENROLL
To enroll in the *Medical Clinics of North America* Continuing Medical Education program, call customer service at 1-800-654-2452 or sign up online at http://www.theclinics.com/home/cme. The CME program is available to subscribers for an additional annual fee of USD $295.

METHOD OF PARTICIPATION
In order to claim credit, participants must complete the following:
1. Complete enrolment as indicated above.
2. Read the activity.
3. Complete the CME Test and Evaluation. Participants must achieve a score of 70% on the test. All CME Tests and Evaluations must be completed online.

CME INQUIRIES/SPECIAL NEEDS
For all CME inquiries or special needs, please contact elsevierCME@elsevier.com.

MEDICAL CLINICS OF NORTH AMERICA

Contributors

CONSULTING EDITORS

DOUGLAS S. PAAUW, MD
Professor of Medicine, Division of General Internal Medicine, Rathmann Family Foundation Endowed Chair for Patient-Centered Clinical Education; Medicine Student Programs, Professor of Medicine, University of Washington School of Medicine, Seattle, Washington

EDWARD R. BOLLARD, MD, DDS, FACP
Professor of Medicine; Associate Dean of Graduate Medical Education, Designated Institutional Official (DIO), Department of Medicine, Penn State–Milton S. Hershey Medical Center, Penn State University College of Medicine, Hershey, Pennsylvania

EDITORS

SUSAN E. MEREL, MD
Assistant Professor, Division of General Internal Medicine, Department of Medicine, University of Washington School of Medicine, University of Washington, Seattle, Washington

JEFFREY WALLACE, MD, MPH, FACP
Professor, Department of Internal Medicine, Division of Geriatric Medicine, University of Colorado School of Medicine, Aurora, Colorado

AUTHORS

CATHY A. ALESSI, MD
Geriatric Research, Education, and Clinical Center, VA Greater Los Angeles Healthcare System, Los Angeles, California; Department of Medicine, David Geffen School of Medicine, University of California

KIRK M. ANDERSON, MD
Fellow in Reconstructive Urology, Division of Urology, Department of Surgery, University of Colorado Denver, Aurora, Colorado

NIDHI BANSAL, MBBS
Department of Medicine, Division of Endocrinology, Diabetes and Metabolism, SUNY Upstate Medical University, Syracuse, New York

DAVID B. BEKELMAN, MD, MPH
Associate Professor, Department of Medicine, Division of General Internal Medicine, University of Colorado School of Medicine, Aurora, Colorado; VA Eastern Colorado Healthcare System, Denver, Colorado

CHARLOTTE CARLSON, MD, MPH
Associate Medical Director, On Lok Senior Health by Institute of Aging, San Francisco, California

SKOTTI CHURCH, MD
Assistant Professor, Division of Geriatric Medicine, University of Colorado School of Medicine, Aurora, Colorado

KARLOTTA DAVIS, MD, MPH
Associate Professor, Department of Obstetrics and Gynecology, Division of Female Pelvic Medicine and Reconstructive Surgery, University of Colorado Denver, Aurora, Colorado

RUBAN DHALIWAL, MD
Assistant Professor, Department of Medicine, Division of Endocrinology, Diabetes and Metabolism, SUNY Upstate Medical University, Syracuse, New York

JOSEPH M. DZIERZEWSKI, PhD
Geriatric Research, Education, and Clinical Center, VA Greater Los Angeles Healthcare System, Los Angeles, California; Department of Medicine, David Geffen School of Medicine, University of California

KARLI EDHOLM, MD
Clinical Instructor, Division of General Internal Medicine, University of Utah School of Medicine, Salt Lake City, Utah

BRIAN J. FLYNN, MD
Associate Professor of Surgery/Urology, Division of Urology, Department of Surgery, University of Colorado Denver, Aurora, Colorado

KERRY L. HILDRETH, MD
Assistant Professor, Division of Geriatric Medicine, University of Colorado School of Medicine, Aurora, Colorado

PHILIP A. KITHAS, MD, PhD
Geriatrics Section Chief, George E. Wahlen Salt Lake Veterans Administration Medical Center; Associate Professor of Medicine, Geriatrics Division, University of Utah School of Medicine, Salt Lake City, Utah

HILLARY D. LUM, MD, PhD
Assistant Professor, Department of Medicine, Division of Geriatric Medicine, University of Colorado School of Medicine, Aurora, Colorado; Department of Medicine, VA Eastern Colorado Healthcare System, Denver, Colorado

JANE E. MAHONEY, MD
Professor of Medicine, Division of Geriatrics and Gerontology, Department of Medicine, University of Wisconsin School of Medicine and Public Health; Executive Director, Wisconsin Institute for Healthy Aging, Madison, Wisconsin

MONICA MALEC, MD
Assistant Professor of Medicine, Section of Geriatrics and Palliative Medicine, University of Chicago, Chicago, Illinois

SUSAN E. MEREL, MD
Assistant Professor, Division of General Internal Medicine, Department of Medicine, University of Washington School of Medicine, University of Washington, Seattle, Washington

DOUGLAS S. PAAUW, MD
Master, American College of Physicians; Rathmann Family Foundation Endowed Chair for Patient-Centered Clinical Education; Division of General Internal Medicine, Professor, Department of Medicine, University of Washington School of Medicine, University of Washington, Seattle, Washington

ELIZABETH A. PHELAN, MD, MS
Associate Professor of Medicine/Gerontology and Geriatric Medicine, Adjunct Associate Professor of Health Services, Harborview Medical Center, Seattle, Washington

NATHAN RAGLE, MD
Clinical Instructor, Division of General Internal Medicine, University of Utah School of Medicine, Salt Lake City, Utah

JUAN CARLOS RODRIGUEZ, MD
Geriatric Research, Education, and Clinical Center, VA Greater Los Angeles Healthcare System, Los Angeles, California; Department of Medicine, David Geffen School of Medicine, University of California, Los Angeles, California; Department of Medicine, Pontificia Universidad Catolica de Chile, Santiago

MATTHEW T. RONDINA, MD, MS
Associate Professor, Program in Molecular Medicine, University of Utah School of Medicine, Salt Lake City, Utah

JOSEPH W. SHEGA, MD
Regional Medical Director, VITAS Healthcare, Miami, Florida

MICHAEL C. SOUNG, MD, FACP
General Internal Medicine, Internal Medicine Residency Core Faculty, Virginia Mason Medical Center, Seattle, Washington

JUDY A. STEVENS, PhD
Epidemiologist, National Center for Injury Prevention & Control, Centers for Disease Control and Prevention, Atlanta, Georgia

REBECCA L. SUDORE, MD
Associate Professor of Medicine, Division of Geriatrics, San Francisco VA Medical Center, University of California, San Francisco, California

MARK A. SUPIANO, MD
D. Keith Barnes, M.D. and Dottie Barnes Presidential Endowed Chair in Medicine, Professor and Chief, Geriatrics Division, University of Utah School of Medicine; Director, VA Salt Lake City Geriatric Research, Education, and Clinical Center; Executive Director, University of Utah Center on Aging, Salt Lake City, Utah

JAN C. VOIT, PT
PT Director, Fall Prevention Clinic; Fall Prevention Specialist, Outpatient Physical and Hand Therapy Clinic, Department of Rehabilitation Medicine, Harborview Medical Center, Seattle, Washington

JEFFREY WALLACE, MD, MPH, FACP
Professor, Department of Internal Medicine, Division of Geriatric Medicine, University of Colorado School of Medicine, Aurora, Colorado

RUTH S. WEINSTOCK, MD, PhD
Department of Medicine, Division of Endocrinology, Diabetes and Metabolism, SUNY Distinguished Service Professor, SUNY Upstate Medical University, Syracuse, New York

MICHI YUKAWA, MD, MPH
San Francisco VA Medical Center, San Francisco, California

Contents

> Deciding when to stop cancer screening in older adults is a complex challenge
> that involves multiple factors: individual health status and life expectancy;
> risks and benefits of screening, which vary with age and comorbidity; and
> individual preferences and values. This article examines current cancer
> screening practices and reviews the risks and benefits of cancer screening
> for colorectal, breast, lung, prostate, and cervical cancer, particularly in older
> individuals and those with multiple comorbidities. Tools for estimating life
> expectancy are reviewed, and a practical framework is presented to guide
> discussions on when the harms of screening likely outweigh the benefits.

> Geriatric assessment is an increasingly important area of outpatient med-
> icine, given the unprecedented aging of the US population. Screening and
> evaluation for geriatric syndromes, particularly falls, urinary incontinence,
> frailty, and cognitive impairment, are crucial aspects of outpatient geriatric
> assessment. Innovative models of care are emerging to improve quality of
> care and enhance cost savings for the geriatric patient. High-value fea-
> tures of geriatric care systems include providing increased 24/7 access
> to care, a multidisciplinary team-based approach to care, performing
> medication reconciliation and comprehensive geriatric assessments, and
> integrating palliative care into treatment planning.

> Falls among older adults are neither purely accidental nor inevitable;
> research has shown that many falls are preventable. Primary care pro-
> viders play a key role in preventing falls. However, fall risk assessment
> and management is performed infrequently in primary care settings. This
> article provides an overview of a clinically relevant, evidence-based
> approach to fall risk screening and management. It describes resources,
> including the STEADI (Stopping Elderly Accidents, Deaths, and Injuries)
> tool kit that can help providers integrate fall prevention into their practice.

Polypharmacy, specifically the overuse and misuse of medications, is associated with adverse health events, increased disability, hospitalizations, and mortality. Mechanisms through which polypharmacy may increase adverse health outcomes include decreased adherence, increased drug side effects, higher use of potentially inappropriate medications, and more frequent drug-drug interactions. This article reviews clinical problems associated with polypharmacy and presents a framework to optimize prescribing for older adults.

Cognitive complaints are common in the geriatric population. Older adults should routinely be asked about any concerns about their memory or thinking, and any cognitive complaint from the patient or an informant should be evaluated rather than be attributed to aging. Several screening instruments are available to document objective impairments and guide further evaluation. Management goals for patients with cognitive impairment are focused on maintaining function and independence, providing caregiver support, and advance care planning. There are currently no treatments to effectively prevent or treat dementia. Increasing appreciation of the heterogeneity of Alzheimer disease may lead to novel treatment approaches.

Persistent pain in older adults is common, and associated with substantial morbidity. Optimal management starts with assessment, including pain presence, intensity, characteristics, and interference; painful conditions; pain behaviors; pain-related morbidity; pain treatments; and coping style. Treatment incorporates analgesics demonstrated to decrease pain and improve a patient's sense of well-being. The World Health Organization's 3-step pain ladder is widely accepted and adopted for selecting analgesics among patients with non-cancer pain. Shared decision making is essential to balance the benefits and burdens of analgesics. This article reviews pain assessment/management for older adults, focusing on commonly used analgesics.

Management of diabetes in the elderly necessitates careful consideration of concomitant geriatric syndromes and comorbid conditions that increase the risk of complications, including severe hypoglycemia. Whereas healthy older adults can use therapeutic approaches recommended for their younger counterparts, treatment plans for frail elderly patients need to be simplified and A_{1c} and blood pressure goals relaxed with the development of impairments in function, cognition, vision, and dexterity. The goals of diabetes management in the elderly should be to maintain quality of life and minimize symptomatic hyperglycemia and drug side effects, including hypoglycemia.

Hypertension contributes greatly to adverse cardiovascular outcomes; the magnitude of this contribution increases with age. The most recent guideline has proposed raising the goal systolic blood pressure to less than 150 mm Hg among those over age 60; however, this recommendation is not endorsed by other organizations. There are multiple contributors to hypertension in the older individual, including increased vascular stiffness, salt sensitivity, and decreased baroreceptor responsiveness. Therapy in the hypertensive patient over age 60 should be individualized and account for patient's health, functional and cognitive status, comorbidities, frailty, and prognosis.

Key components of advance care planning (ACP) for the elderly include choosing a surrogate decision maker, identifying personal values, communicating with surrogates and clinicians, documenting wishes in advance directives, and translating values and preferences for future medical care into medical orders. ACP often involves multiple brief discussions over time. This article outlines common benefits and barriers to ACP in primary care, and provides practical approaches to integrating key ACP components into primary care for older adults. Opportunities for multidisciplinary teams to incorporate ACP into brief clinic visits are highlighted.

Urinary incontinence and pelvic organ prolapse are widely prevalent in the elderly population. The primary care physician should play a leading role in identifying the presence of incontinence in this population, as it can significantly affect quality of life and well-being. Behavioral and lifestyle modification is the cornerstone in treatment and can be initiated in the primary care setting. Frail elderly require special consideration to avoid potentially serious complications of urinary incontinence and pelvic organ prolapse.

Older patients with atrial fibrillation have an increased risk of stroke and systemic embolism compare with younger patients. For most patients, oral anticoagulation remains the most effective way to reduce this risk. Although vitamin K antagonists have been used for decades, the more recent development of non-vitamin K–dependent oral anticoagulants provides clinicians with a broader selection of anticoagulants for stroke prevention in older patients with AF. This article discusses stroke risk-stratification tools for clinical decision making, reviews pharmacologic options for the prevention of stroke, and highlights several practical considerations to the use of these agents in older adults.

Epidemiologic studies have shown that approximately 50% of older adults have sleep problems, many of which carry deleterious consequences that affect physical and mental health and also social functioning. However, sleep problems in late life are often unrecognized, and are inadequately treated in clinical practice. This article focuses on the diagnosis and treatment of the 2 most common sleep problems in older patients: sleep apnea and insomnia.

Foreword

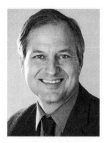

Douglas S. Paauw, MD, MACP
Consulting Editor

The majority of patients in an internist's practice are over the age of 65. A deep and workable understanding of geriatrics is crucial for all internists, whether practicing in the inpatient or outpatient setting. In this issue of *Medical Clinics of North America*, Drs Merel and Wallace have put together a practical, useful set of topics that help guide us to better care of our geriatric patients. The nuances of appropriate assessment, prescribing, and goals of care in this growing patient population are covered well. As internists, we need to recognize that diseases are not always treated the same way in different patient populations, especially in our geriatric population. The articles on diabetes, hypertension, insomnia, and cancer screening are excellent examples of this important geriatric principle. More is often less in the care of our geriatric patients. More medications, more invasive tests, and more specialists may not lead to better outcomes. This issue does an excellent job of helping guide us on the narrow path of excellent care for our geriatric patients.

Douglas S. Paauw, MD, MACP
Rathmann Family Foundation Endowed Chair for Patient-Centered Clinical Education
Division of General Internal Medicine
Department of Medicine
University of Washington School of Medicine
Seattle, WA 98195, USA

E-mail address:
DPaauw@medicine.washington.edu

Med Clin N Am 99 (2015) xv
http://dx.doi.org/10.1016/j.mcna.2014.12.002
0025-7125/15/$ – see front matter © 2015 Published by Elsevier Inc.

Preface

Toward Improving the Care of Older Adults

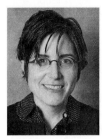 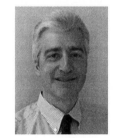

Susan E. Merel, MD   Jeffrey Wallace, MD, MPH, FACP
Editors

Beautiful young people are accidents of nature, but beautiful old people are works of art.

—*Eleanor Roosevelt*

In this era of evidence-based medicine, the practice of geriatric medicine stands out as an area whereby guidelines are often not easily applied. Sometimes this is due to a lack of evidence because clinical trials only rarely include frail, medically complex, or very old persons. Other times, evidence pertinent to the patient's issue at hand is available, but the application is complicated due to guidelines that may be overlapping or conflicting and may not match the care preferences of an older adult with multiple medical and psychosocial problems. Following guidelines designed for younger adults can even lead to harm in the elderly, for example, when strict blood pressure control contributes to falls. The aging of the Baby Boomers creates the imperative that all generalists be prepared for the challenges inherent in caring for older adults. We must be prepared to move past simple application of guidelines to an approach to the older patient that minimizes disability and maximizes quality of life.

This issue of *Medical Clinics of North America* considers important issues in the care of older adults with a focus on providing approaches to optimizing care of elderly persons with common and challenging conditions. Geriatricians are taught a syndromes-based, holistic approach to the patient encounter that strives to reduce disability and align care with the patient's social situation and goals. This conceptual framework is essential in developing an approach to the care of the elderly patient. Authors review important aspects of this approach in articles about geriatric syndromes and assessment, cancer screening in older adults, and polypharmacy and rational prescribing. Tools to help assess prognosis, promote discussion of patient care preferences, and complete advance directives are provided.

Med Clin N Am 99 (2015) xvii–xviii
http://dx.doi.org/10.1016/j.mcna.2014.12.001
0025-7125/15/$ – see front matter © 2015 Published by Elsevier Inc.

medical.theclinics.com

Next, we have attempted to review specific issues that primary providers face every day when caring for older adults. Key aspects of geriatric medicine and overarching problems such as evaluating cognitive concerns and managing pain are reviewed. The use of newer medications and application of guidelines pertinent to specific medical conditions are considered in articles devoted to diabetes, hypertension, urinary incontinence, sleep disorders, and anticoagulation in atrial fibrillation in older adults.

It is our hope that the articles contained herein will provide new information and insights to help primary care providers enhance their care of older adults. We are grateful to the outstanding group of educators and clinicians who have contributed articles to this effort.

Susan E. Merel, MD
Division of General Internal Medicine
Department of Medicine
University of Washington School of Medicine
1959 NE Pacific Street
Box 356429
Seattle, WA 98195-6429, USA

Jeffrey Wallace, MD, MPH, FACP
Department of Internal Medicine
Division of Geriatric Medicine
University of Colorado School of Medicine
Mail Stop B179
12631 E. 17th Avenue, Room 8111
Aurora, CO 80045, USA

E-mail addresses:
smerel@uw.edu (S.E. Merel)
jeff.wallace@ucdenver.edu (J. Wallace)

Erratum

The article "Glycemic Targets: What is the Evidence?" by Silvio Inzucchi and Sachin Majumdar (Med Clin N Am 2015;99:47-67) was published with the incorrect reference attributed to Figure 6 (page 51). The Figure 6 legend should read: "CV events according to HbA₁c in the European Prospective Investigation of Cancer (EPIC)-Norfolk study. (*Data from* Khaw K, Wareham N, Bingham S, Luben R, Welch A, Day N. Association of Hemoglobin A1c with Cardiovascular Disease and Mortality in Adults: The European Prospective Investigation into Cancer in Norfolk. Ann Intern Med. 2004;141:413-420.)" The authors apologize for the error.

Med Clin N Am 99 (2015) xix
http://dx.doi.org/10.1016/j.mcna.2015.01.001
0025-7125/15/$ – see front matter © 2015 Elsevier Inc. All rights reserved.

Screening for Cancer: When to Stop?

A Practical Guide and Review of the Evidence

Michael C. Soung, MD

KEYWORDS

- Cancer screening • Elderly • Life expectancy • Breast cancer • Colorectal cancer
- Lung cancer • Prostate cancer • Cervical cancer

KEY POINTS

- Decisions about when to stop cancer screening should consider life expectancy, risks and benefits (which vary with age and comorbidity), and individual values.
- A practical method starts by categorizing individuals into general categories of health (eg, below average, average, above average).
- These estimations should be based on easily accessible measures such as gait speed, comorbidity, and functional status. Validated prognostic indices can also be helpful.
- For women of below average, average, and above average health, consider stopping breast and colorectal cancer screening around ages 70, 80, and 85 years; stop a few years earlier in men.

INTRODUCTION

Cancer screening is a cornerstone of preventive health care. For screening to be effective, it must detect cancer in a preclinical phase, before the cancer becomes clinically apparent, during which treatment is more beneficial.[1] In order to achieve a mortality benefit from screening, a person must have sufficient life expectancy and be healthy enough to tolerate the treatments associated with a cancer diagnosis. Although there is reasonable consensus as to the appropriate age to start screening for various cancers, there is considerably less clarity as to when screening is no longer likely to be beneficial. The decision to stop screening should be based on multiple factors, including age, health status, patient preferences, and the risks and benefits associated with screening.

This review examines current cancer screening practices, as well as the risks and benefits of cancer screening, with a focus on health status and older age. It also

---

Disclosures: The author has no relevant disclosures.
General Internal Medicine, Internal Medicine Residency Core Faculty, Virginia Mason Medical Center, 1100 Ninth Avenue, Seattle, WA 98101, USA
E-mail address: michael.soung@vmmc.org

Med Clin N Am 99 (2015) 249–262
http://dx.doi.org/10.1016/j.mcna.2014.11.002   **medical.theclinics.com**
0025-7125/15/$ – see front matter © 2015 Elsevier Inc. All rights reserved.

proposes a practical framework to guide discussions on when the harms of screening likely outweigh the benefits.

CURRENT SCREENING PRACTICES

Current cancer screening guidelines (**Table 1**) provide little or conflicting advice on when to discontinue screening. Cervical cancer screening is the exception; there is good consensus that this can be stopped at age 65 years, or after a woman has undergone a total hysterectomy for benign purposes. For other cancers, the guidelines vary, with some providing cutoffs based on either age or life expectancy, or no specific cutoff.

There is good consensus that the benefits of cancer screening are delayed. Effective screening generally detects cancers or precancers years before they would have been lethal. Screening people who would have died of another cause exposes them to the harms of the screening process and subsequent treatment without extending their lives. For breast cancer, benefits of screening seem to be delayed at least 3 to 10 years.[18–20] For cervical[19] and colorectal cancer,[2,20–22] estimates range from at least 4 to 10 years, and for prostate cancer the time period seems to be at least 7 to 10 years.[1,23,24] Lung cancer screening may have a shorter lag time to benefit.[25]

Recent data suggest that a substantial portion of cancer screening is being done in patients who are unlikely to benefit. One cross-sectional population-based study of Papanicolaou (Pap) smears found that that nearly two-thirds of women aged 65 years or older reported recent Pap screening, including 45% of the women in that age group who had previously undergone a hysterectomy.[26] Another study of mammography and Pap smears showed that more than half of women aged 80 years or older in the worst health quartile had undergone recent screening.[27] Screening rates decreased with age but not with worsening health status. A Veterans Affairs study of colorectal cancer screening in veterans aged 70 years or older showed that those with severe comorbidities had a screening rate of 41%, despite a 5-year mortality of 55%.[28] This finding compared with a screening rate of 47% in veterans with no comorbidity, whose 5-year mortality was just 19%. Screening rates for colorectal cancer decreased with age but varied little with worsening health status. In addition, a cross-sectional study of prostate-specific antigen (PSA) screening found that more than 30% of older men with life expectancies of 5 years or less had recent PSA screening.[29]

Why so much screening? One public survey found that 87% of respondents thought that routine cancer screening is almost always a good idea and that 30% to 40% thought it would be irresponsible for an 80-year-old to decline cancer screening.[30] An interview study of older adults being seen at a senior health center reflected this view that undergoing screening was morally obligatory.[31] Physician interviews suggest that discussions about stopping screening can be uncomfortable and time consuming and it would useful to have more data to guide these discussions.[32]

EVIDENCE FOR CANCER SCREENING IN THE ELDERLY
Colorectal Cancer Screening

Randomized controlled trials (RCTs) of fecal occult blood testing have included more than 40,000 people aged 70 to 80 years. Colorectal cancer mortality is reduced by 15% to 20%, and this effect is independent of age.[19] Among RCTs of flexible sigmoidoscopy,[33–36] only 1 has included adults older than age 64 years. More than 50,000 participants aged 65 to 74 years had a 35% reduction in colorectal cancer mortality (vs 16% in younger adults).[36] The remaining evidence for lower endoscopy in older

Table 1
Selected guidelines on when to discontinue cancer screening

Colorectal Cancer	Breast Cancer	Lung Cancer	Prostate Cancer	Cervical Cancer
USPSTF (2008)[2]: Age 76–85 y: against routine screening, consider in individual patients Age>85 y: against screening	USPSTF (2009)[6]: Age≥75 y: insufficient evidence	USPSTF (2013)[9]: Screen until age 80 y, or if >15 y since last smoked, or health problem that substantially limits life expectancy or the ability or willingness to have curative lung surgery	USPSTF (2012)[12]: Against screening at any age	USPSTF (2012)[16]: Age>65 y
ACS (2008)[3]: No recommendation on stopping age	ACS (2003)[7]: Stop if life expectancy <3–5 y, severe functional limitations, and/or multiple or severe comorbidities likely to limit life expectancy	ACS (2013)[10]: Age>74 y or >15 y since last smoked, as along as in "relatively good health"	ACS (2010)[13]: Consider if life expectancy ≥10 y	ACS (2012)[10]: Age>65 y
ASCE (2006)[4]: No recommendation on stopping age	ACOG (2011)[8]: Age≥75 y: consider medical comorbidity and life expectancy	ACCP (2013)[11]: Age>74 y, >15 y since last smoked, or "severe comorbidities that would preclude potentially curative treatment and/or limit life expectancy"	AUA (2013)[14]: Age≥70 y or life expectancy <10–15 y ("some men age 70+ y in excellent health may benefit from...screening")	ACOG (2012)[17]: Age>65 y
ACP (2012)[5]: Age>75 y, or life expectancy <10 y[31]			ACP (2013)[15]: Age>69 y or life expectancy <10–15 y	All assume adequate recent screening; ie, ≥2–3 consecutive normal Pap smears in the past 10 y and no history of cervical intraepithelial neoplasia 2 or higher. Also consensus on stopping if total hysterectomy for a benign indication

Abbreviations: ACCP, American College of Chest Physicians; ACOG, American Congress of Obstetricians and Gynecologists (formerly American College of Obstetricians and Gynecologists); ACP, American College of Physicians; ACS, American Cancer Society; ASCE, American Society for Gastrointestinal Endoscopy; AUA, American Urological Association; Pap, Papanicolaou; USPSTF, US Preventive Services Task Force.

adults is mostly limited to case-control trials, which included subjects aged 70 to 91 years. Screening with lower endoscopy is associated with 60% lower colorectal cancer mortality, again independent of age.[19]

However, the absolute benefits of colorectal cancer screening wane with age. A cross-sectional study of 1244 consecutive patients undergoing screening colonoscopy suggested that patients aged 80 years and older had a much smaller gain in life expectancy than patients aged 50 to 54 years (0.13 years vs 0.85 years).[37] The benefit seems to decrease even more dramatically with worsening health status, as shown by a cohort study of Medicare patients.[38] An otherwise healthy woman diagnosed with stage I colorectal cancer at age 75 years has a life expectancy of more than 15 years from diagnosis. If she were 81 years old but still otherwise healthy at diagnosis, her life expectancy would be 14 years. However, at age 75 years but with at least 3 chronic health conditions, her life expectancy would be just 5 years. As a result, she would be unlikely to live long enough to realize a benefit from screening. Similar patterns were seen in men.

In contrast, the harms of colorectal cancer screening increase with age and comorbidity. Another cohort study of Medicare patients aged 66 to 95 years undergoing colonoscopy showed a low overall risk of bowel perforation: 0.6 per 1000 procedures. However, the risk of serious gastrointestinal (GI) adverse events was 75% higher for subjects aged 80 to 84 years compared with those aged 66 to 69 years. The risk for GI adverse events was similarly increased in those with certain comorbid conditions: diabetes, stroke, chronic obstructive pulmonary disease, atrial fibrillation, and congestive heart failure.[39]

Breast Cancer Screening

RCTs of screening mammography have shown a reduction in breast cancer mortality only in women aged 69 years and younger. No RCTs enrolled patients older than 74 years, and there has been no benefit shown in the small numbers of women aged 70 to 74 years included in these trials.[6] There are some observational data suggesting benefit from screening mammography in older women. In one study of older women with breast cancer, mammographic detection was associated with a 50% lower risk of death in women aged 80 years and older who had no more than 1 comorbid condition. However, there was no significant benefit seen in women aged 75 years and older who had 2 or more comorbid conditions.[40] Other observational trials on mammography have generally shown similar results.[41]

The harms of screening mammography in older women are also not well defined. Modeling studies estimate 2 fewer breast cancer deaths for every 1000 women aged 70 to 79 years undergoing screening mammography. However, 200 women would experience false-positive mammograms and, more concerning, 13 women would be overdiagnosed (ie, diagnosed with a cancer that never would have become clinically relevant in that person's lifetime). Overdiagnosis exposes people to the harms of treatment without the benefits. Moreover, the harms of breast cancer treatment, including surgery, chemotherapy, radiotherapy, and posttreatment prophylaxis, are increased in older women and in those with limited life expectancy.[41]

Lung Cancer Screening

The largest RCT of lung cancer screening using low-dose computed tomography (LDCT) was limited to participants up to the age of 74 years.[25] Included were ~14,000 people aged 65 to 74 years; about one-quarter of the total population studied. Fewer than 10% were aged 70 to 74 years. Overall, LDCT reduced lung cancer mortality by 20% more than 6.5 years, and all-cause mortality by 7%. This benefit seems to be independent of age.[42] However, the trial excluded those with medical conditions that posed a substantial risk for death during the 8-year trial and those who were unlikely to complete curative lung cancer surgery. As a result, the population studied was unusually healthy, and it has been noted that people with comorbid conditions may experience substantially less net benefit, or even net harm.[9]

Lung cancer screening is associated with significant harms. After 3 rounds of screening, 24.2% of screening tests were positive, and 96.4% of these were false-positives.[9] In the modeling study that led the US Preventive Services Task Force to recommend screening up to age 80 years, it was predicted that for every 19,300 persons screened there would be 67,550 false-positive screens, 910 procedures for benign lesions, and 190 cases of overdiagnosis, with 497 lung cancer deaths averted.[43] The risk for overdiagnosis, about 10% overall, increases with age and worsening health status.[44] False-positive results, complications from biopsy of pulmonary nodules, and postoperative mortality from resection of nodules all worsen with age. On April 30, 2014, the Medicare Evidence Development & Coverage Advisory Committee gave a vote of low confidence about whether the benefits of LDCT screening would outweigh the harms among Medicare beneficiaries in a community setting.[45] However, on November 10, 2014, the Centers for Medicare & Medicaid Services released a proposed decision memo supporting the use of LDCT in Medicare beneficiaries.[46] At the time of this writing, the decision was still in the public comment phase. National guidelines generally recommend screening only in settings that can deliver an organized, comprehensive lung cancer screening program.[9–11]

Prostate Cancer Screening

PSA-based prostate cancer screening remains controversial, although there is some consensus that screening should be discontinued at age 70 years,[14,15] if performed at all. There have been 5 RCTs of PSA screening, all of poor to fair quality.[47] The 2 largest trials have had conflicting results. One trial studied men aged 55 to 74 years and showed no reduction in prostate cancer mortality after 13 years of follow-up, although there were high rates of PSA screening in the control group.[48] The other showed a 21% reduction in prostate cancer mortality with PSA screening after 13 years.[24] A related substudy of men aged 50 to 64 years showed a greater benefit at 14 years of follow-up.[23] The overall trial included men up to age 74 years at entry, although the benefit was limited to men younger than 70 years of age. In addition, RCTs of prostatectomy for early-stage prostate cancer have not shown a reduction in prostate cancer mortality in men more than 65 years old.[49,50]

The harms of prostate cancer screening in older men have not been directly assessed but can be inferred from RCTs in younger men. Overdiagnosis is a major concern, with wide-ranging estimates of 5% to 75%, and the risk increases with age.[14] In PSA-screened men aged 50 to 74 years followed for 13 years, 27 need to be diagnosed with prostate cancer to prevent 1 prostate cancer death.[24] Risks of prostate cancer treatment include urinary incontinence and erectile dysfunction. False-positive PSAs occur in 12% to 13% of men undergoing 3 to 4 rounds of screening.[47] In contrast, autopsy studies suggest very high rates of clinically unimportant prostate cancer. One-third of men aged 40 to 60 years have histologically evident prostate cancer; that proportion increases to three-fourths of men older than 85 years. However, the lifetime risk of dying from prostate cancer is 2.8%.[12]

Cervical Cancer Screening

There is good consensus that cervical cancer screening should be stopped at age 65 years in women who have had adequate recent screening, or following a total hysterectomy for benign purposes. Modeling studies suggest that screening beyond age 65 years provides a small (<1 life-year) benefit but increases potential harms because of false-positive results and resultant colposcopies and biopsies.[16] Fewer than 1 in 1000 women older than 60 years with a normal baseline Pap smear develops high-grade cervical lesions or cervical cancer. This risk is nearly doubled in women without previous Pap smears. More than 80% of women with high-grade cervical lesions or cancer had either abnormal or no Pap smears.[18] One study of 9610 vaginal Pap smears in women who had undergone a total hysterectomy for benign purposes showed an abnormal Pap smear rate of 1.1% but no cases of vaginal or cervical cancer.[51]

ESTIMATING LIFE EXPECTANCY

Life expectancy is a critical factor in the decision to stop screening. However, the wide variability in health status and life expectancy in older individuals poses a difficult challenge. There are several published models for estimating life expectancy in community-dwelling patients.[52] Two prognostic indices (by Lee and colleagues[53] and Schonberg and colleagues[54]) have been published that use brief questionnaires based on patient self-report to predict 4-year or 5-year life expectancy. Both models incorporate age, sex, body mass index (BMI; BMI<25 in older individuals is associated with lower life expectancy), comorbid conditions (including diabetes mellitus, chronic lung disease, history of cancer, smoking), and a few functional measures (eg, ability to walk several blocks and manage everyday needs). The models have since been further validated to estimate 9-year and 10-year life expectancy.[55,56] These and other prognostic calculators can be accessed online at www.eprognosis.org. Another population-based cohort study quantified the effect of comorbidity on a Medicare population. Categorizing people based on degree of comorbidity (none, low/medium, high) made it possible to make life expectancy estimations. Those with low/medium comorbidity had predicted life expectancies close to average for age, whereas those with no or high comorbidity had life expectancies that were 3 to 10 years longer or shorter.[57]

A recent pooled analysis of cohort studies also showed the predictive value of gait speed, in combination with age and sex, in estimating life expectancy (**Fig. 1**). The standard measurement is a walk at usual pace from a standing start over a distance of 4 m (13.1 feet). The gait speed associated with median life expectancy is 0.8 m/s, or 4 m in 5 seconds. Faster gait speeds (eg, 1.3 m/s, or 4 m in 3 seconds) are associated with above average life expectancies. Slower gait speeds (eg, 0.4 m/s, or 4 m in 10 seconds), are associated with shorter life expectancies.[58]

WHAT DO PATIENTS WANT?

Some providers may be uncomfortable initiating discussions on whether or not to continue cancer screening. However, some data suggest that older adults look to their physicians to raise these issues. One study of adults aged 70 years and older in independent living retirement communities showed that 84% of residents wanted their doctors to talk with them about whether to stop getting tests to check for cancer. Of these residents, 94% wanted to hear about limitations of cancer screening and 52% wanted to discuss life expectancy to help them with cancer screening decisions.[59] Another study in older women found that the number 1 factor influencing their decision to undergo screening mammography was their doctor's recommendation.[60] Discussions involving the balance of risks and benefits, as well test burdens and complications, may be more effective than those focused on the role of statistics and/or recommendations of government panels.[31]

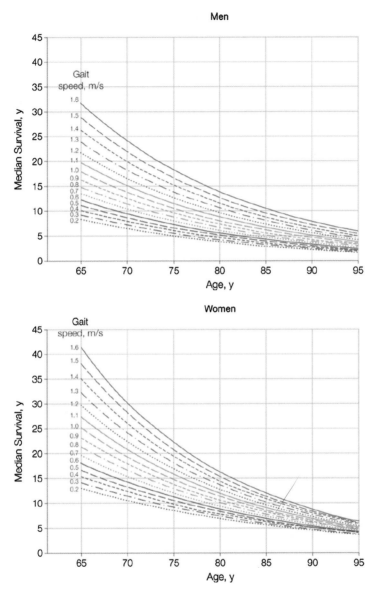

Fig. 1. Gait speed and survival in older adults. (*From* Studenski S, Perera S, Patel K, et al. Gait speed and survival in older adults. JAMA 2011;305(1):54; with permission.)

PUTTING IT ALL TOGETHER: A PRACTICAL APPROACH (OR 70, 80, 85 YEARS)

In 2001, Walter and Covinsky[21] proposed a thoughtful framework to help individualize cancer screening decisions in older adults. They calculated numbers needed to screen for different cancers at various ages and life expectancy quartiles to help guide personalization of cancer screening recommendations. In this context, I propose a practical method for estimating the ages after which individuals are unlikely to benefit from further breast and colorectal cancer screening, based on the assumptions noted in **Box 1**.

Box 1

Key assumptions for estimating cessation ages for cancer screening

- Benefits of screening decrease with age and comorbidity
- Harms of screening increase with age and comorbidity
- Benefits of cancer screening are delayed, typically at least 3 to 10 years
- Harms are likely to outweigh the benefits when life expectancy is less than 10 years
- Prognostic models are inexact and there is always individual variation
- Individual patient values and preferences need to play a major role
- Clinicians might benefit from a quick guide to personalize cancer screening recommendations

---

The first step is to categorize whether a person's health is below average, average, or above average (**Box 2**). This categorization may be simpler and more palatable than estimating a life expectancy for individual patients. Prognostication is an inexact science but some of the tools described earlier can be used to get a general sense of an individual's health status. The aforementioned prognostic indices suggest that clinicians should consider the number of comorbidities (including diabetes mellitus, chronic lung disease, history of cancer, smoking), a person's functional status (ability to walk several blocks and manage everyday needs), and a person's BMI (<25 in older individuals is associated with lower life expectancy). Low BMI, each individual comorbidity, and each functional measure are given roughly equal weight. As a general guide, patients with 3 or more of these factors could be characterized as having below average life expectancy. Having none of these factors would indicate above average life expectancy, whereas 1 to 2 factors would be considered average. As an example, a 72-year-old woman with BMI of less than 25, chronic lung disease, and difficulty walking several blocks (3 factors) has an estimated 10-year mortality of 52% based on the Lee Index, indicating below average life expectancy. Even more simply, a brief observation of gait speed could be used to help stratify people into general categories of health, as described earlier.

These health estimates can then be used to determine a recommended stopping age for breast and colorectal cancer screening. Using a life expectancy of less than

---

Box 2

Proposed approach to estimating stopping ages for breast and colorectal cancer screening

1. Categorize health status as below average, average, or above average, based on[a]:

   - Gait speed (based on 4-m walk: 10 seconds = below average, 5 seconds = average, 3 seconds = above average [see text for more details])
   - Comorbidity (eg, diabetes mellitus, chronic lung disease, history of cancer, smoking)
   - Functional status (eg, ability to walk several blocks, ability to manage everyday needs)
   - BMI<25 in older adults is associated with lower life expectancy

2. Consider the following stopping ages for below average, average, and above average health status: 70, 80, 85 years for women (a few years younger for men)

[a] Gait speed can be used as a standalone measure. For the other measures, consider adding up the total number of individual factors: 0, above average; 1 to 2, average; 3, below average health. Some patients may be interested in more specific predictions of their 4-year and 10-year mortalities; these prognostic calculators as well as others can be accessed at www.eprognosis.org.

10 years as a general cutoff, the following age guidelines can be determined for women with below average, average, or above average health: 70, 80, and 85 years, respectively (**Fig. 2**). In other words, a woman in average health is unlikely to benefit from breast or colorectal cancer screening after the age of 80 years. A woman in below average health is unlikely to benefit after the age of 70 years.

To clarify, this is not to suggest that all women be screened all the way up to these stopping ages. Personal preferences might prompt them to stop screening at a younger age. In contrast, there may be rare individuals with exceptionally good health that might, for example, reasonably be screened past the age of 85 years. Individual preferences and values must play a critical role in these discussions. However, given that the benefits of screening decrease with age and worsening health, whereas the harms from screening increase with age and worsening health, I propose that these ages roughly estimate the ages after which women are more likely to be harmed than to benefit from screening.

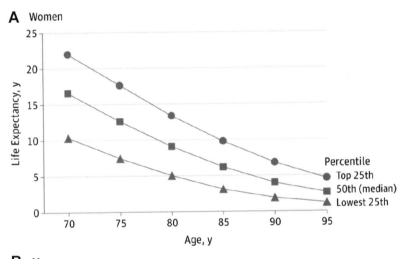

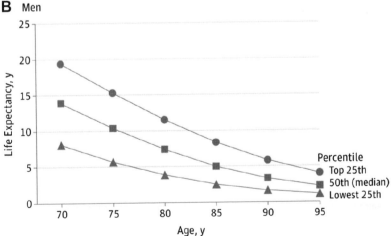

Fig. 2. Upper, middle, and lower quartiles of life expectancy at selected ages. (*From* Walter LC, Schonberg M. Screening mammography in older women: a review. JAMA 2014;331:1341; with permission.)

Men have shorter life expectancies than women (see **Fig. 2**). Thus, corresponding age guidelines for colorectal cancer screening in men are a few years younger than for women. For prostate cancer screening, the situation is more complicated because there is still controversy over weighing benefits from screening versus the risks of overdiagnosis, overtreatment, and false-positive testing at any age. Reductions in prostate cancer mortality in RCTs have been limited to men less than 70 years of age, and screening is unlikely to benefit men with a life expectancy of less than 10 years.

This general approach has support from a recent modeling study that estimated the harms and benefits of breast, colorectal, and prostate cancer screening by age and comorbid conditions.[61] The study simulated screenings in persons with no, mild, moderate, or severe comorbidity at various ages. Compared with an average health 74-year-old, screening results were similar for those with no, mild, moderate, or severe comorbidity until ages 76, 74, 72, and 66 years. The investigators noted that their model overestimates the life expectancy for patients with worse comorbidity and underestimates the life expectancy for those with less comorbidity, so this age spread may be even wider than suggested. Also noted are rates of overdiagnosis for prostate cancer estimated at 15 to more than 100 times greater for prostate cancer versus breast or colorectal cancer screening. For lung cancer screening, similar morbidity-stratified data are not available. However, the same general concepts likely apply.

SUMMARY

Cancer screening in older adults represents a complex challenge that requires accounting for multiple factors: individual health status and life expectancy; risks and benefits of screening, which vary with age and comorbidity; and individual preferences and values.

- For cervical cancer screening, there are clear guidelines on stopping at age 65 years (assuming recent normal Pap smears) or following a hysterectomy for benign purposes.
- For prostate cancer screening, there is controversy over the risk-benefit analysis at any age, although benefits seem to be limited to men younger than 70 years with life expectancy of greater than 10 years.
- For breast and colorectal cancer screening, I propose using easily accessible measures of health status (such as gait speed, comorbid conditions, functional status, BMI) to categorize individuals into below average, average, or above average health, and to consider discontinuation of screening no later than ages 70, 80, and 85 years for women (a few years younger for men).
- For lung cancer, a stopping age of 74 to 80 years has been recommended; however, patients with significant comorbidity are unlikely to benefit.

I hope that this framework can help guide an informed discussion of the risks and benefits of cancer screening in the context of each individual's preferences and values.

REFERENCES

1. Balducci L. Prevention of cancer in the older person. Cancer J 2005;11:442–8.
2. US Preventive Services Task Force. Screening for colorectal cancer: U.S. Preventive Services Task Force recommendation statement. Ann Intern Med 2008;149: 627–37.

3. Levin B, Lieberman DA, McFarland B, et al. Screening and surveillance for the early detection of colorectal cancer and adenomatous polyps, 2008: a joint guideline from the American Cancer Society, the US Multi-Society Task Force on Colorectal Cancer, and the American College of Radiology. CA Cancer J Clin 2008;58:130–60.
4. ASGE Standards of Practice Committee. ASGE guideline: colorectal cancer screening and surveillance. Gastrointest Endosc 2006;63:546–57.
5. Qaseem A, Denberg TD, Hopkins RH. Screening for colorectal cancer: a guidance statement from the American College of Physicians. Ann Intern Med 2012;156:378–86.
6. US Preventive Services Task Force. Screening for breast cancer: U.S Preventive Services Task Force recommendation statement. Ann Intern Med 2009;151:716–26.
7. Smith RA, Saslow D, Sawyer KA, et al. American Cancer Society guidelines for breast cancer screening: update 2003. CA Cancer J Clin 2003;53:141–69.
8. American College of Obstetricians-Gynecologists. Practice bulletin no. 122: breast cancer screening. Obstet Gynecol 2011;118:372–82.
9. Moyer VA, on behalf of the USPSTF. Screening for lung cancer: US Preventive Services Task Force recommendation statement. Ann Intern Med 2014;160:330–8.
10. Smith RA, Brooks DB, Cokkinides V, et al. Cancer screening in the United States, 2013. CA Cancer J Clin 2013;63:87–105.
11. Detterbeck FC, Mazzone PJ, Naidich DP, et al. Screening for lung cancer: diagnosis and management of lung cancer, 3rd ed: American College of Chest Physicians evidence-based clinical practice guidelines. Chest 2013;143(5 Suppl):e78S–92S.
12. Moyer VA, on behalf of the USPSTF. Screening for prostate cancer: U.S. Preventive Services Task Force recommendation statement. Ann Intern Med 2012;157:120–34.
13. Wolf AM, Wender RC, Etzioni RB, et al. American Cancer Society guideline for the early detection of prostate cancer: update 2010. CA Cancer J Clin 2010;60:70.
14. Carter HB, Albertsen PC, Barry MJ, et al. Early detection of prostate cancer: AUA guideline. American Urological Association; 2013.
15. Qaseem A, Barry MJ, Denberg TD, et al. Screening for prostate cancer: a guidance statement from the Clinical Guidelines Committee of the American College of Physicians. Ann Intern Med 2013;158:761–9.
16. Moyer VA, on behalf of the USPSTF. Screening for cervical cancer: U.S. Preventive Services Task Force recommendation statement. Ann Intern Med 2012;156:880–91.
17. Committee on Practice Bulletins—Gynecology. ACOG practice bulletin number 131: screening for cervical cancer. Obstet Gynecol 2012;120:1222–38.
18. Albert RH, Clark MM. Cancer screening in the older patient. Am Fam Physician 2008;78:1369–74, 1376.
19. Walter LC, Lewis CL, Barton MB. Screening for colorectal, breast, and cervical cancer in the elderly: a review of the evidence. Am J Med 2005;118:1078–86.
20. Lei SJ, Boscardin WJ, Stijacic-Cenzer I, et al. Time lag to benefit after screening for breast and colorectal cancer: meta-analysis of survival data from the United States, Sweden, United Kingdom, and Denmark. BMJ 2012;345:e8441.
21. Walter LC, Covinsky KE. Cancer screening in elderly patients. JAMA 2001;285:2750–6.

22. Lewis CL, Griffith J, Pignone MP, et al. Physicians' decisions about continuing or stopping colon cancer screening in the elderly: a qualitative study. J Gen Intern Med 2009;24:816–21.

23. Hugosson J, Carlsson S, Aus G, et al. Mortality results from the Goteborg randomised population-based prostate-cancer screening trial. Lancet Oncol 2010; 11:725–32.

24. Schroder FH, Hugosson J, Roobol MJ, et al. Screening and prostate cancer mortality: results of the European Randomised Study of Screening for Prostate Cancer (ERSPC) at 13 years of follow-up. Lancet 2014. http://dx.doi.org/10.1016/S0140-6736(14)60525-0.

25. The National Lung Screen Trial Research Team. Reduced lung-cancer mortality with low-dose computed tomographic screening. N Engl J Med 2011;365:395–409.

26. Watson M, King J, Ajani U, et al. Cervical cancer screening among women by hysterectomy status and among women aged ≥65 years – United States, 2000-2010. MMWR Morb Mortal Wkly Rep 2013;61:1043–7.

27. Walter LC, Lindquist K, Covinsky KE. Relationship between health status and use of screening mammography and Papanicolaou smears among women older than 70 years of age. Ann Intern Med 2004;140:681–8.

28. Walter LC, Lindquist K, Nugent S, et al. Impact of age and comorbidity on colorectal cancer screening among older veterans. Ann Intern Med 2009;150:465–73.

29. Drazer MW, Huo D, Schonberg MA, et al. Population-based patterns and predictors of prostate-specific antigen screening among older men in the United States. J Clin Oncol 2001;29:1736–43.

30. Schwartz LM, Woloshin S, Fowler FJ, et al. Enthusiasm for cancer screening in the United States. JAMA 2004;291:71–8.

31. Torke AM, Schwartz PH, Holtz LR, et al. Older adults and forgoing cancer screening. JAMA Intern Med 2013;173:526–31.

32. Schonberg MA, Ramanan RA, McCarthy EP, et al. Decision making and counseling around mammography screening for women aged 80 or older. J Gen Intern Med 2006;21:979–85.

33. Hoff G, Grotmol T, Skovlund E, et al. Risk of colorectal cancer seven years after flexible sigmoidoscopy screening: randomized controlled trial. BMJ 2009;338:b1846.

34. Atkin WS, Edwards R, Kralj-Hans I, et al. Once-only flexible sigmoidoscopy screening in prevention of colorectal cancer: a multicenter randomised controlled trial. Lancet 2010;375:1624–33.

35. Segnan N, Armaroli P, Bonelli L, et al. Once-only sigmoidoscopy in colorectal cancer screening: follow-up findings of the Italian Randomized Controlled Trial–SCORE. J Natl Cancer Inst 2011;103:1310–22.

36. Schoen RE, Pinsky PF, Weissfeld JL, et al. Colorectal-cancer incidence and mortality with screening flexible sigmoidoscopy. N Engl J Med 2012;366:2345–57.

37. Lin OS, Kozarek RA, Schembre DB, et al. Screening colonoscopy in very elderly patients. JAMA 2006;295:2357–65.

38. Gross CP, McAvay GJ, Krumholz HM, et al. The effect of age and chronic illness on life expectancy after a diagnosis of colorectal cancer: implications for screening. Ann Intern Med 2006;145:646–53.

39. Warren JL, Klabunde CN, Mariotto AB, et al. Adverse events after outpatient colonoscopy in the Medicare population. Ann Intern Med 2009;150:849–57.

40. McPherson CP, Swenson KK, Lee MW. The effects of mammographic detection and comorbidity on the survival of older women with breast cancer. J Am Geriatr Soc 2002;50:1061–8.

41. Walter LC, Schonberg M. Screening mammography in older women: a review. JAMA 2014;331:1336–47.
42. Pinsky PF, Church TR, Ismirlian G, et al. The National Lung Screening Trial: results stratified by demographics, smoking history, and lung cancer histology. Cancer 2013;119:3976–83.
43. De Koning HJ, Meza R, Plevritis SK, et al. Benefits and harms of computed tomography lung cancer screening strategies: a comparative modeling study for the US Preventive Services Task Force. Ann Intern Med 2014;160:311–20.
44. Humphrey LL, Deffebach M, Pappas M, et al. Screening for lung cancer with low-dose computed tomography: a systematic review to update the US Preventive Services Task Force Recommendation. Ann Intern Med 2013;159:411–20.
45. Wiener RS. Balancing the benefits and harms of low-dose computed tomography screening for lung cancer: Medicare's options for coverage. Ann Intern Med 2014. http://dx.doi.org/10.7326/M14-1352. Available at: www.annals.org. Accessed June 24, 2014.
46. Centers for Medicare and Medicaid services (CMS). Proposed Decision Memo for Screening for Lung Cancer with Low Dose Computed Tomography (LDCT) (CAG-00439N). Available at: http://www.cms.gov/medicare-coverage-database/details/nca-proposed-decision-memo.aspx?NCAId=274.
47. Chou R, Croswell JM, Dana T, et al. Screening for prostate cancer: a review of the evidence for the US Preventive Services Task Force. Ann Intern Med 2011;155:762–71.
48. Andriole GL, Crawford ED, Grubb RL, et al. Prostate cancer screening in the randomized prostate, lung, colorectal, and ovarian cancer screening trial: mortality results after 13 years of follow-up. J Natl Cancer Inst 2012;104:125–32.
49. Bill-Axelson A, Holmberg L, Garmo H, et al. Radical prostatectomy or watchful waiting in early prostate cancer. N Engl J Med 2014;370:932–42.
50. Wilt TJ, Brawer MK, Jones KM, et al. Radical prostatectomy versus observation for localized prostate cancer. N Engl J Med 2012;367:203–13.
51. Pearce KF, Haefner HK, Sarwar SF, et al. Cytopathological findings on vaginal Papanicolaou smears after hysterectomy for benign gynecologic disease. N Engl J Med 1996;335:1559–62.
52. Yourman LC, Lee SJ, Schonberg MA, et al. Prognostic indices for older adults: a systematic review. JAMA 2012;307:182–92.
53. Lee SJ, Lindquist K, Segal MR, et al. Development and validation of a prognostic index for 4-year mortality in older adults. JAMA 2006;295:801–8.
54. Schonberg MA, Davis RB, McCarthy EP, et al. Index to predict 5-year mortality of community-dwelling adults aged 65 and older using data from the National Health Interview Survey. J Gen Intern Med 2009;24:1115–22.
55. Schonberg MA, Davis RB, McCarthy EP, et al. External validation of an index to predict up to 9-year mortality of community-dwelling adults aged 65 and older. J Am Geriatr Soc 2011;59:1444–51.
56. Cruz M, Covinsky K, Widera EW, et al. Predicting 10-year mortality for older adults. JAMA 2013;309:874–6.
57. Cho H, Klabunde CN, Yabroff KR, et al. Comorbidity-adjusted life expectancy: a new tool to inform recommendations for optimal screening strategies. Ann Intern Med 2013;159:667–76.
58. Studenski S, Perera S, Patel K, et al. Gait speed and survival in older adults. JAMA 2011;305:50–8.
59. Lewis CL, Kistler CE, Amick HR, et al. Older adults' attitudes about continuing cancer screening later in life: a pilot study interviewing residents of two continuing care communities. BMC Geriatr 2006;6:10.

60. Schonberg MA, McCarthy MA, York M, et al. Factors influencing elderly women's mammography screening decisions: implications for counseling. BMC Geriatr 2007;7:26.
61. Lansdrop-Vogelaar I, Gulati R, Mariotto AB, et al. Personalizing age of cancer screening cessation based on comorbid conditions: model estimates of harms and benefits. Ann Intern Med 2014;161:104–12.

Geriatric Syndromes and Geriatric Assessment for the Generalist

 CrossMark

Charlotte Carlson, MD, MPH[a],*, Susan E. Merel, MD[b],
Michi Yukawa, MD, MPH[c]

KEYWORDS

- Geriatric syndromes • Geriatric assessment • Frailty • Care delivery systems
- Primary care

KEY POINTS

- It is crucial to recognize geriatric syndromes, multifactorial conditions occurring primarily in the elderly, in the primary care setting.
- The most important geriatric syndromes to recognize in primary care are falls, urinary incontinence, frailty, and cognitive impairment.
- Elements of ideal geriatric primary care include assessment of functional status, frequent medication review, careful evaluation of the benefits and burdens of any new test or treatment, and frequent assessment of goals of care and prognosis.
- Innovative delivery systems, such as the GRACE, PACE, and Hospital-at-Home models, can improve geriatric primary care. High-value features of geriatric care systems include ensuring 24/7 access to care, providing a team-based approach to care, performing medication reconciliation and comprehensive geriatric assessments, and integrating palliative care into treatment planning.

INTRODUCTION

With an unprecedented growth of the aging population anticipated in the next century, understanding the health needs and demands of older adults is of crucial importance for the future of the US health care system. By 2050, 1 of every 5 people living in the United States will be 65 or older.[1] As more Americans are living longer, the practicing generalist clinician will need to use geriatric principles, tools, and approaches in his or her everyday work.

---

[a] On Lok Senior Health by Institute of Aging, 3575 Geary Boulevard, San Francisco, CA 94118, USA; [b] Division of General Internal Medicine, Department of Medicine, University of Washington, 1959 NE Pacific Street, Box 356429, Seattle, WA 98195, USA; [c] San Francisco VA Medical Center, 4150 Clement St, San Francisco, CA 93121, USA
* Corresponding author.
E-mail address: Charlotte.carlson@ucsf.edu

Med Clin N Am 99 (2015) 263–279
http://dx.doi.org/10.1016/j.mcna.2014.11.003
0025-7125/15/$ – see front matter © 2015 Elsevier Inc. All rights reserved.

What is different about caring for an older adult? As a group, older adults have increased rates of comorbidity, experience unique age-related physiologic changes, and are more prone to iatrogenic illness than younger adults.[2] Most older adults have at least one chronic disease, if not multiple diseases, and substantial numbers will have impairments in abilities to perform basic and instrumental activities of daily living.[3] The US elderly population is also heterogeneous, and many people in the older than 65 age group are healthy, health conscious, and infrequent users of health care.

Geriatric assessment is a multifaceted approach that focuses on understanding the physical, cognitive, psychological, and social domains of an individual older adult. A crucial component of geriatric assessment includes the screening and evaluation for geriatric syndromes. Geriatric syndromes acknowledge the complex interplay between age-related physiologic changes, chronic disease, and functional stressors in older adults. The approach to managing key geriatric syndromes in the outpatient setting (falls, cognitive impairment, incontinence, and frailty) is outlined in this article, and tools for the practicing clinician to diagnose and treat geriatric syndromes in the office visit also are provided.

Coordinating a comprehensive plan for a complex geriatric patient across multiple health care settings is a challenging task, and often requires fundamental system redesign to improve quality and coordination of care. As care of an older adult often extends across a variety of care settings, including hospital, ambulatory clinic, rehabilitation center, and community-based long-term care settings, geriatric care delivery is complex, and depends on coordination of multiple providers. As an introduction to geriatric care system design, this article outlines high-value system features of geriatric care, and describes examples of current geriatric care models.

GERIATRIC SYNDROMES, FUNCTIONAL STATUS, AND THE FRAIL ELDERLY PATIENT IN PRIMARY CARE

A geriatric syndrome is a multifactorial condition that involves the interaction between identifiable situation-specific stressors and underlying age-related risk factors, resulting in damage across multiple organ systems.[4] Geriatric syndromes have a devastating effect on the individual's quality of life as they progress, may lead to significant disability, and are part of the "cascade to dependency" that can often result in institutionalization.[5,6] An elderly patient whose chief complaint is a result of a geriatric syndrome will often present with symptoms that are difficult to attribute to the organ system causing the initial pathology. The geriatric syndromes most relevant to those caring for older adults in the outpatient setting are falls, cognitive impairment, incontinence, and frailty.

Clinicians should attempt to treat or manage a geriatric syndrome even though a single cause may not be able to be identified. Whereas in a younger person a workup may look primarily for single diseases, the interaction of multiple physiologic changes and comorbidities in an older adult warrant a broader perspective. Diagnostic testing that would be relevant in a younger person may not be as beneficial in an older person, and/or may lead to unnecessary treatment and/or harm for the patient. For example, in the case of a fall, although an echocardiogram would be a likely part of the diagnostic workup for a younger individual to rule out cardiac syncope, in an older adult, pursuing an echocardiogram may be more likely to result in abnormalities that may lead to unnecessary further diagnostic testing. **Box 1** further illustrates the difference between a traditional medical approach and the geriatric approach to a fall.

Geriatric syndromes overlap with common aging-related risk factors. In a population-based cohort of community-dwelling elderly patients with falls,

---

Box 1
Comparison of traditional medical approach and geriatric approach to a syndrome, using falls as an example

Traditional Medical Approach

Diagnosis and Treatment

1. Extensive search for cause of falls in most patients (eg, cardiac monitoring and echocardiogram, neurologic workup with imaging if indicated, tilt-table testing)

2. Medical treatments directed at likely causes (eg, rate control for atrial fibrillation, pacemaker for bradycardia, medical treatment for peripheral neuropathy)

Geriatric Approach

Risk Factor Assessment and Reduction

1. More limited search for medical cause of falls in some patients (eg, cardiac monitoring only for clearly syncopal falls and only if treatment of cardiac condition would be within goals of care)

2. More limited set of medical treatments if a clear medical cause of falls is found

3. Assess for risk factors for multifactorial mechanical falls and target interventions toward eliminating risk factors (eg, strength training for leg weakness, training in use of assistive device for transfers if falls occur during transfers, home safety evaluation by occupational therapist, and installation of lights at home if falls triggered by inadequate lighting).

Adapted from Labella AM, Merel SE, Phelan EA. Ten ways to improve the care of elderly patients in the hospital. J Hosp Med 2011;6:362; with permission.

---

incontinence, and functional dependence, Tinetti and colleagues[7] found 4 independent predisposing factors: upper and lower extremity weakness, decreased vision and hearing, and anxiety or depression. Similarly, Inouye and colleagues[8] performed a systematic review of studies identifying risk factors for pressure ulcers, incontinence, falls, functional decline, and delirium and found that older age, functional impairment, cognitive impairment, and impaired mobility were shared risk factors. Interventions may be effective in preventing some of these shared risk factors and therefore managing more than one geriatric syndrome. For example, strategies for management of delirium also may reduce falls, and Tai Chi may be helpful in preventing both falls and cognitive decline.[9,10]

Frailty is an important concept in geriatrics and has been described as "the overarching geriatric syndrome" due to its importance in predicting treatment benefit and prognosis (**Fig. 1**).[5] There are a number of subtly different definitions of frailty

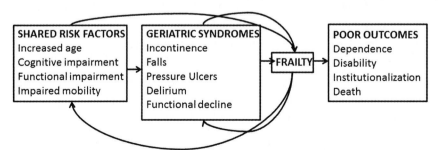

Fig. 1. The relationship between risk factors, geriatric syndromes and poor outcomes. (*Adapted from* Inouye SK, Studenski S, Tinetti ME, et al. Geriatric syndromes: clinical, research, and policy implications of a core geriatric concept. J Am Geriatr Soc 2007;55:782; with permission.)

used in geriatric research, but the definition most relevant to the practicing clinician is a clinical syndrome including 3 or more of the following: unintentional weight loss, self-reported exhaustion, weakness, slow walking speed, and/or low physical activity (**Box 2**).[11] Fried and colleagues[11] showed that the frailty phenotype in elders followed over a 3-year period is independently predictive of incident falls, disability, hospitalization, and death. Furthermore, frail elders are at an increased risk for developing other geriatric syndromes.[5] Identifying frailty in a patient often can change the trajectory of care, because it implies a more limited life expectancy and increased disease burden.

Evaluation of functional status is an important component of geriatric assessment and should be part of routine geriatric care. Functional impairment, defined as a limitation on a person's ability to perform basic tasks, such as bathing or dressing, may be the first harbinger of a geriatric syndrome. For example, a study of preclinical disability in community-dwelling older adults with normal cognition and mild cognitive impairment (MCI) suggested that inability to perform 2 specific instrumental activities of daily living (IADLs), shopping and balancing one's checkbook, correctly classified 80% of the cohort as having MCI; difficulty with these 2 IADLs was more accurate in discriminating those with normal cognition from those with MCI than Mini-Mental State Examination (MMSE) scores or depressive symptoms.[12] Conversely, specific conditions that are commonly discovered as part of evaluation for geriatric syndromes, such as extremity weakness, depression, and vision and hearing loss, are predictors of future functional decline both on their own and as part of a geriatric syndrome (eg, a patient with hearing loss may be at increased risk for falls and also may develop functional disability related specifically to the hearing loss, such as the inability to use a telephone to complete his or her IADLs).[13]

Evaluating functional status, frailty, and other geriatric syndromes while simultaneously addressing individual disease processes is at the heart of geriatric approach to primary care (**Fig. 1**). Switching from a single disease framework to a broader holistic approach, as outlined in **Boxes 3** and **4**, helps tailor care planning to the individual patient and maximizes the overall treatment benefit. Studies have found that using a geriatric approach that focuses on functional assessment improves ability of a patient to comply with the treatment plan and helps prevent adverse drug events.[14] Furthermore, developing a comprehensive assessment of the geriatric patient helps to guide decision-making and incorporate patient preferences into decisions, helping patients and families evaluate whether evidence-based treatments will truly benefit a specific older adult.[15]

Box 2
Definition of frailty

A clinical syndrome including 3 or more of the following:

1. Unintentional weight loss of more than 10 lb in the previous year

2. Self-reported exhaustion

3. Weakness (as measured by grip strength in the lowest 20% by gender and body mass index)

4. Slow walking speed (in the lowest 20% by gender and height)

5. Low physical activity (as measured by kcal/wk in the lowest 20%)

Note: this is a definition for research purposes and cannot be measured precisely in the clinic setting, but provides a helpful framework.
Adapted from Fried LP, Tangen CM, Walston J, et al. Frailty in older adults: evidence for a phenotype. J Gerontol A Biol Sci Med Sci 2001;56:M148; with permission.

Box 3
Ten ways to optimize primary care for the frail elderly in the traditional primary care setting

1. Learn to quickly identify frail elderly patients; they are most vulnerable to adverse outcomes and most benefit from a holistic geriatric approach

2. Be aware of common geriatric syndromes, including falls, delirium/cognitive impairment, functional dependence, and urinary incontinence and consider them in every patient

3. Familiarize yourself with efficient assessment tools for geriatric syndromes; teach nonphysician staff to administer them when possible

4. Be familiar with community resources, such as fall prevention programs, PACE programs, and senior centers

5. Consider a patient's goals, life expectancy, and functional status before considering any test or procedure

6. Review advanced directives and goals of care periodically

7. Familiarize yourself with the Beers Criteria, use it to identify potentially inappropriate medications in the elderly and perform comprehensive medication review periodically

8. Adopt an evidence-based approach to health screening in the frail elderly

9. Have a high suspicion for mood disorders in the frail elderly and consider using geriatric-specific screening tools, such as the 5-item Geriatric Depression Scale

10. Provide caregiver support when possible.

Adapted from American Geriatrics Society 2012 Beers Criteria Update Expert Panel. American Geriatrics Society updated Beers criteria for potentially inappropriate medication use in older adults. J Am Geriatr Soc 2012;60:616–31; and Hoyl MT, Alessi CA, Harker JO, et al. Development and testing of a five-item version of the geriatric depression scale. J Am Geriatr Soc 1999;47:873–8.

A PRACTICAL APPROACH TO THE ASSESSMENT OF SPECIFIC GERIATRIC SYNDROMES

A complete assessment of geriatric syndromes often requires an interprofessional team approach, which may not be readily available in the typical outpatient practice. However, there are evaluation tools that can be performed relatively quickly that are just as effective in diagnosing geriatric syndromes. A brief approach to screening of the 4 most common geriatric syndromes, falls, cognitive impairment, urinary incontinence, and frailty, are addressed in the following sections.

Falls

Approximately one-third of community-dwelling adults older than 65 have 1 fall per year.[16] Some risk factors for falls can be modified, whereas others cannot be improved.[17] The American Geriatrics Society and the British Geriatrics Society developed a fall prevention algorithm that can be easily used for fall assessment (**Fig. 2**).[18] A comprehensive fall evaluation requires an interprofessional team approach, but the initial assessment can be performed in primary care clinics. Simple tests, such as the Get Up and Go and Functional Reach Tests, can be done in less than a minute and can provide accurate risk for falls (**Table 1**).[19–23] A thorough physical examination should include a vision test and a thorough examination of the patient's feet and shoes. Laboratory tests may include a complete blood count to rule out significant anemia, a chemistry panel to rule out electrolyte abnormalities, and Vitamin B12 and 25-OH Vitamin D levels. After the clinician has completed the falls assessment, he or she should consider simple evidence-based interventions, including referral to a physical therapist for balance and strengthening exercises and occupational

> **Box 4**
> **Suggested approach to the evaluation and management of the older adult with multimorbidity**
>
> Based on recommendations of the American Geriatrics Society Expert Panel on the Care of Older Adults with Multimorbidity
>
> 1. Inquire about the patient's and/or caregiver's primary concern and/or objectives for visit.
> 2. Conduct a complete review of the care plan for the person with multimorbidity OR focus on a specific aspect of care.
> 3. What are the current medical conditions and interventions? Is there adherence/comfort with the treatment plan?
> 4. Consider patient preferences.
> 5. Is relevant evidence available regarding important outcomes?
> 6. Consider the patient's prognosis.
> 7. Consider interactions within and among treatments and conditions.
> 8. Weigh benefits and harms of components of the treatment plan.
> 9. Communicate and decide for or against implementation or continuation of intervention/treatment.
> 10. Reassess at selected intervals for benefit, feasibility, adherence, and alignment with preferences.
>
> *Adapted from* American Geriatrics Society Expert Panel on the Care of Older Adults with Multimorbidity. Patient-centered care for older adults with multiple chronic conditions: a stepwise approach from the American Geriatrics Society. J Am Geriatr Soc 2012;60:1958; with permission.

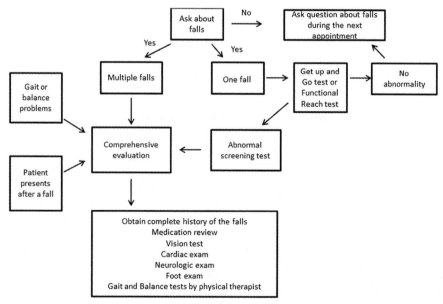

Fig. 2. Falls assessment algorithm. (*Adapted from* Panel on Prevention of Falls in Older Persons, American Geriatrics Society and British Geriatrics Society. Summary of the updated American Geriatrics Society/British Geriatrics Society clinical practice guideline for prevention of falls in older persons. J Am Geriatr Soc 2011;59:150.)

Table 1
Assessment tools for falls/gait abnormality

Assessment Tools for Falls	Brief Description
Performance-Oriented Mobility Assessment	Patient is asked to perform a series of maneuvers that test the quality of transfer, balance, and gait (ie, sitting balance, rising from a chair, standing balance, 1-leg balance, balance with eyes closed). Each movement is rated as normal, adaptive, or abnormal.[19]
Short Physical Performance Battery	Tests of standing balance (tandem, semitandem and side-by-side stands). Test of walking speed (8-foot walking speed). Test of ability to get up from a chair with arms across the chest.[20]
Berg Balance Test	14-item test including sitting to standing, standing unsupported, sitting unsupported, transfers, standing with eyes closed, reaching forward with an outstretched arm, and so forth. Each task is scored from 0–4. Maximum score is 56 and score <45 imply increased risk for falls.[21]
Get Up and Go	Patient is asked to get up from an armchair without using his or her hands. Then patient walks across the room (3 m) and turns and walks back to the chair and sits down. If this test takes >13.5 s to complete then he or she is at risk for future falls.[22]
Functional Reach Test	Patient is asked to stand perpendicular and close to a wall with arms forward. Then ask the patient to extend the arm forward as far as possible without losing balance to taking a step. Measure the difference in arm stretch from standing to the reached position. If the functional reach is <10 inches then he or she has increased risk for falling.[23]

therapists for home safety evaluation; collaboration with a pharmacist to review and adjust medications; and ophthalmology evaluation.

Cognitive Impairment

Cognitive impairment and dementia are conditions feared by older adults and their families because of chronic, debilitating decline, resulting in loss of personality and independence. Dementia is common, with a prevalence of dementia of 5% for adults aged 71 to 79 and 24% for a person between the ages of 80 and 89. For adults older than 90 years, dementia prevalence rate is 37%.[24]

The most commonly used screening tests for cognitive impairment are listed in **Table 2**. Whereas the MMSE is the most commonly used test for research purposes,

Table 2
Screening tests for cognitive impairment

Tests	Description
MMSE	30-item test that is copyright protected. Need to adjust for age and level of education. Score ≤24 is considered abnormal.
Montreal Cognitive Assessment (MoCA)	30-item test that has been validated in multiple languages. It is not copyright protected. It can be downloaded free at www.mocatest.org. Score of ≤26 is considered abnormal.[26]
Mini-cog	Clock-drawing test and 3-item recall. If both are normal, then rule out cognitive impairment. If either one is abnormal, then screen in as cognitive impairment.[27]

it is copyright protected. However, the MoCA and Mini-cog tests may be used freely in the clinic, and are just as sensitive and specific in screening for cognitive deficit as the MMSE.[25–28]

Laboratory tests should be ordered to rule out potentially reversible causes such as metabolic abnormalities (hypothyroidism, hypercalcemia, or hyperglycemia), rapid plasma reagin (RPR) to rule out syphilis, and Vitamin B12 levels.[28] The yield of a head computed tomography (CT) scan or MRI for evaluation of cognitive impairment remains controversial, especially in a patient without neurological abnormalities. However, if no neuroimaging has been conducted recently, a noncontrast head CT scan or MRI can be obtained to evaluate for normal-pressure hydrocephalus, subdural hematoma, or tumor.[28]

Diagnosing patients with cognitive impairment or dementia is paramount in guiding clinical care and arranging for adequate social support. Advanced care planning becomes crucial, as dementia often progresses to limit the capacity of patients to understand risks and benefits of important medical and social decisions. Ideally, clinicians should discuss a patient's preference for end-of-life care and establish a health care proxy or durable power of attorney at diagnosis of MCI or mild dementia. Home safety and driving issues should be also addressed. In some states, clinicians are mandated to report moderate and severe dementia patients to the Department of Motor Vehicles, and older adults with MCI or mild dementia may need to take a special test annually to keep their driver's license. For patients with moderate dementia, focus should remain on safety, particularly risk for wandering and getting lost, behavior disturbance, and, importantly, assess for caregiver burden or stress. For patients with severe dementia, providers should shift the care to maximizing comfort and quality of life.

URINARY INCONTINENCE

Urinary incontinence (UI) occurs in approximately 15% to 30% of healthy community-dwelling older adults. UI is frequently underreported because of the patient's embarrassment to discuss this with the physician and some misconception that it is part of normal aging. UI can be divided broadly into 2 categories: acute or reversible UI and chronic UI. Potential causes of acute UI include infection, atrophic vaginitis, delirium, psychological disorder, reduced mobility, excess urine output, stool impaction, and medications.[29] Common causes of chronic UI are listed in **Table 3**.[28] Although chronic UI is more commonly encountered in older adults, some may develop acute UI, and thus evaluation for reversible causes of UI is warranted.

As with all geriatric syndromes, a thorough history of UI is the foremost step in assessment. A voiding diary to document timing, circumstances and severity of UI, amount of urine leaked, potential triggers, and frequency of UI is very helpful for

Table 3	
Categories of chronic urinary incontinence	
Types	**Symptoms**
Stress	Loss of urine with increased abdominal pressure, after cough, laughing, or straining.
Urge	Detrusor overactivity and feeling of frequent urge to urinate.
Mixed	Usually a combination of stress and urge incontinence.
Overflow	Overdistended bladder, which leads to frequent leakage of urine.
Functional	Urinary incontinence in a setting of normal function of urinary tract. Inability to access the toilet, commode, or urinal in time.

clinicians and patients.[28] **Table 4** outlines screening tools that can be used to quickly identify UI in the clinic.[30–33] A thorough review of all medications, including over-the-counter medications, is essential in excluding pharmaceutical causes of UI. Physical examination should include a cardiac examination to rule out congestive heart failure, abdominal examination to evaluate for distended bladder or abnormal mass, and rectal examination to assess prostate size or abnormal mass and rectal tone to rule out spinal cord or neuropathic dysfunction. Gynecologic examination in women should be performed if physically possible to assess for organ prolapse, vaginal atrophy, or uterine/pelvic mass. Simple laboratory tests, such as urinalysis and urine culture to rule out infection, and electrolytes to evaluate renal function and rule out metabolic causes are sufficient.

FRAILTY

As discussed previously, frailty is often thought of as the overarching geriatric syndrome, given its impact across disease states and great impairments in function. Approximately 5% of Americans older than 60 have been diagnosed with frailty.[34] Frailty can change a treatment trajectory, most commonly by increasing the impact of physical stress during acute medical illness or surgery. Several studies have shown that preoperative frailty is associated with higher postoperative complications after

Table 4	
Screening tools for urinary incontinence	
Tool	**Description**
The 3 Incontinence Questions (Brown et al,[31] 2006)	1. During the past 3 mo, have you leaked urine? If the answer is yes, then complete the rest of the questionnaire. 2. During the past 3 mo, did you leak urine: when you were performing some physical activity? Without physical activity? When you had the urge to urinate, could you get to the toilet fast enough? 3. During the past 3 mo, did you leak urine most often: when you were performing some physical activity? Without physical activity? When you had the urge to urinate, could you get to the toilet fast enough?
American Urologic Association BPH Symptom Score Index (Barry et al,[32] 1995)	During the past month: How often did you feel you did not empty your bladder fully? How often did you have to urinate within 2 h? How often did you have to stop and restart urination? How often did you find it difficult to delay urination? How often did you notice a weak urinary stream? How often did you have to push and strain to start urination? How often did you have to urinate at night? Likert scale of 0–5: 0 = not at all and 5 = almost always
Overactive Bladder Validated 8 Question Awareness Tool (Coyne et al,[33] 2005)	How much have you been bothered by the following: Frequent daytime urination? Uncomfortable urge to urinate? Sudden urge to urinate? Loss of small amount of urine? Uncontrollable urge to urinate? Urine loss due to strong desire to urinate? Nighttime urination? Waking up at night to urinate? Likert scale of 0–5: 0 = not at all and 5 = bothered a very great deal

Data from Refs.[31–33]

colorectal and cardiac surgery than nonfrail or prefrail patients.[35,36] Similarly, frail patients had longer hospital stays and higher 30-day readmission rates postoperatively than nonfrail or prefrail individuals.[35,36] Patients with chronic renal failure and frailty had increased risk of mortality than those without frailty.[37] Frail patients experiencing an acute coronary syndrome had longer hospital stay, decreased procedure use, and increased mortality compared with nonfrail patients.[38] Given the close relationship between frailty and treatment outcome, early recognition of frailty is paramount in guiding clinical care and discussing future procedures with patients and their families.

In 2001, several predictive scales were introduced to define and characterize frailty. Frailty index (FI) was defined using the data from the Canadian Study of Health and Aging. The original 92 items included physical symptoms and signs, functional impairments, and laboratory abnormalities, and since then various versions of the FI have been developed and tested to predict morbidity and mortality.[39,40] The formula for determining the FI is included in **Table 5**. High FI scores have been shown to be highly correlated with mortality, but obtaining all the information on FI is not very practical in a busy outpatient clinic practice.[41] The Frail phenotype was developed and operationalized in the Cardiovascular Health Study.[11] It is based on 5 items, but some characteristics are not easily ascertained from patients, such as grip strength and estimation of their activity levels (see **Table 5**). The FRAIL and Study of Osteoporotic Fractures Frailty Scale are easier to administer (see **Table 5**).[42–45]

Several studies have compared and contrasted these frailty scales and they found all of them to be effective in predicting mortality among community-dwelling older adults.[41,44,45] Therefore, the FRAIL and Study of Osteoporotic Fracture Frailty scales, which are easier to perform than the other frailty scales, are the recommended instruments for use in a clinic setting.

GERIATRIC CARE SYSTEMS: INNOVATIVE CARE DELIVERY FOR THE COMPLEX PATIENT
Contrasting Complex Geriatric Care Needs with Usual Primary Care Needs

Complex geriatric patients have different care needs than most primary care patients. Unlike patients with intermittent, acute problems, complex geriatric patients have multiple chronic diseases and daily symptoms, and frequently require services from different practitioners in the hospital, home, community, and outpatient settings. Because of frequent care needs, geriatric patients have high utilization of health care services and are among the most costly patients in the health care system.[46,47]

The most influential determinant of cost and complexity in geriatric medicine is functional disability. Patients with chronic conditions in combination with limitations on their ability to perform basic daily functions due to physical, mental or psychosocial challenges account for twice the average of Medicare spending.[48] Functional limitations are accompanied by a need for assistance by others to perform routine activities of life, and thus require ongoing long-term services and supports.[48]

Because of a need for ongoing long-term supports, episode-based care delivery systems often do not provide enough opportunity for complex geriatric patients to access care. As complex patients require frequent coordination and comprehensive assessments, planned visits become important approaches to care. Instead of focusing only on acute complaints, these assessments place an emphasis on identifying early complications and prevention of functional decline. Complex geriatric patients are heterogeneous in disease severity and presentation and require integration of functional status and prognosis into care planning. Because of this heterogeneity, available treatment options differ. Personal values and priorities become an essential part of determining care plans for complex geriatric patients.

Table 5 Frailty index scales		
Name of Scale	**Descriptions**	**Scale**
FI[39]	92 items[6] $$FI=\frac{\text{Number of health deficits present}}{\text{Number of health deficits measured}}$$	Score range from Frail score >0.25, prefrail score 0.25–0.2
Frail phenotype–based Cardiovascular Health Study[42]	Weight loss $\geq$10 pounds unintentionally in 12 mo Grip strength: lowest 20% Exhaustion: self-report Slow walking time/15 feet (by gender and height) Low activity: Men <383 kcal/wk Women <270 kcal/wk	Score range from 0–5 Frail score 3–5, prefrail score 1–2
FRAIL (Fatigue, Resistance, Ambulation, Illness, Loss of Weight)[43]	Fatigue: How much time during the past 4 wk they felt tired. 1 point if they answered most of the time or all the time. Resistance: They had any difficulty walking up 10 steps alone without rest or assistance. One point if they answered yes. Ambulation: Whether they had any difficulty walking several hundred yards alone and without aids. One point if they answered yes. Illness: scored 1 point if they reported $\geq$5 illness Loss of weight: scored 1 point if $\geq$5% weight loss within past 12 mo.	Score range from 0–5 Frail score 3–5, prefrail score 1–2
Study of Osteoporotic Fractures Frailty Scale[44]	Weight loss >5% in the past 12 mo Inability to get up from a chair 5 times without using the arms Negative answer to "do you feel full of energy?"	Score range from 0–3 Frail score 2–3, prefrail score 1

Data from Refs.[39,42–44]

Features of Complex Care Delivery Models That Provide Value to Geriatric Patients

Complex geriatric patients are at the center of reform efforts to improve care and control cost, and a number of programs to improve care for complex geriatric patients have been developed in recent years. The high-performing models of complex care delivery share 5 core features (**Table 6**). First, systems that provide complex geriatric patients 24/7 access to their medical team have found higher patient satisfaction with care and lower emergency department use.[49,50] Having 24/7 access allows for discovery of symptoms early in a chronic disease course, thus preventing unnecessary hospitalization. Continuity with a primary care provider has been found to be associated with reductions in mortality, and evidence suggests that night and weekend access is crucial to improving quality of care for complex geriatric patients.

Second, an interdisciplinary team-based approach to care that includes more than one discipline is important for ensuring coordination of care for complex geriatric patients. Although there is no standard composition of team structure, most models

Table 6 High-value features of geriatric care delivery models	
Feature	Description/Rationale
24/7 Access to care	Allows for discovery of symptoms early in chronic disease course
Team-based approach	Multidisciplinary team improves coordination and increases patient engagement
Medication reconciliation	Prevents adverse events during care transitions
Comprehensive assessment	Self-management tools and caregiving support can improve engagement in plan and smooth transitions in care
Integration of palliative care	Helps improve quality of life and align care with patient and family goals

include a registered nurse (RN) and social worker.[51,52] The most effective models use intensive case management and rely on smaller caseloads to ensure quality coordination of care.[50,53]

Third, performing medication reconciliation after transitions in care, particularly after a hospitalization, can improve quality of care and aid in coordination for complex geriatric patients.[54] Medication-related discrepancies are common when patients transition from hospital to home health care. For example, in one large cohort study, 14% of 65-year-old or older community-dwelling adults experienced 1 or more medication discrepancy after discharge.[55] Randomized trials have found that care transition interventions involving RN-pharmacist or pharmacist visits help to resolve issues with transition and reduce adverse events and rehospitalization.[56–58]

Fourth, performing comprehensive geriatric assessments, which combine medical, social, and behavioral aspects of care into treatment planning, can improve quality and efficiency of care.[59] Comprehensive geriatric assessment commonly includes medication management, vision, mobility, fall assessment, and home safety. Assessments are then used to develop individualized care plans to tailor the care services to the patient.

Finally, delivery systems that integrate palliative care into planning for complex patients increase patient satisfaction and decrease utilization of care.[60,61] The most relevant aspects of palliative care medicine for complex geriatric patients are quality-of-life assessment, symptom management, advance care planning, and attention to family experiences in care.[62] Providing support for caregivers in the form of respite care also is an important feature of high-performing geriatric models of care.

Examples of Geriatric Care Systems

Programs to improve delivery of care for complex geriatric patients vary widely in design, target population, and goals. Successful care models can be generally classified into 3 categories: comprehensive programs that provide all medical and social care, consultant-based programs that work in partnership with primary care teams, and short-term interventions that target transitions in care (**Table 7**).

Comprehensive, community-based geriatric systems are designed to provide nursing home–level care in a home or community (ie, adult day center) setting. These programs integrate inpatient, outpatient, and long-term care services, and coordinate all medical and social aspects of care. The Program of All-Inclusive Care of the Elderly (PACE) is an example of a Medicare-funded system that provides comprehensive care services to community-dwelling frail adults.[63] To qualify for a PACE program, a person must be at least 55 years of age and eligible for care in a nursing home. PACE

Table 7
Examples of geriatric care models

Model Type	Description	Example
Comprehensive models	Provides comprehensive care, including hospital, home care, respite care, and personal care	Program for All-Inclusive Care for the Elderly (PACE)[64,65]
Consult models	Provides added geriatric team (often nurse practitioner and/or social worker) as consultants to primary care practice	Geriatric Resources for Assessment and Care for Elders (GRACE)[52]
Short-term models	Targets transitions in care (ie, from hospital to skilled nursing facility or from hospital to home) or provides short-term hospital-level care at home	Hospital-at-Home Model[68] Care Transitions Model[55]

programs revolve around the provision of medical and social services by an interdisciplinary team. Much of the care is delivered at an adult day center.[64] Compared with the general Medicare population, PACE participants spend fewer days in the hospital, and sustain greater function and independence at home.[63]

Another model type involves adding geriatric consultants to primary care teams. A consultant-type approach allows primary care teams to tailor services to a patient's specific medical and social needs. In these models, nurse practitioners and/or social workers often are used to coordinate care, and provide comprehensive geriatric assessment and symptom monitoring in-home settings. An example of a home-based coordinated model is Geriatric Resources for Assessment and Care of Elders (GRACE), which integrates home visits by nurse practitioners alongside primary care teams.[65] GRACE was shown to improve social and mental health measures, and reduce emergency room visits, in a population of low-income older patients.[66]

Finally, instead of comprehensive care or consulting assessment, geriatric care interventions can involve short-term interventions, such as providing hospital-level care for acute conditions at home, or providing intensive short-term transitional care at hospitals. One example of a short-term in-home model is Hospital-at-Home, which provides hospital-level care for older home-limited adults for conditions such as cellulitis, chronic heart failure exacerbation, or pneumonia. The Hospital-at-Home model has been shown to reduce per-patient costs with increase in patient satisfaction and similar quality standards to hospital care.[67,68] Among the transition models targeting complex patients at discharge from hospitals, models described by Naylor and colleagues[69] and Coleman and colleagues[55] have both reduced costs by avoiding unnecessary readmissions or prolonged skilled nursing home stays. Successful features of these interventions include frequent in-home assessment and coordination with primary care teams to identify gaps in care and improve response to added support if needed.

FUTURE CONSIDERATIONS

As the population ages, the complexity of older patients will increase the demands on the US health care system. Because of national shortages of geriatricians, there is an increasing need for generalists to have knowledge of geriatric principles, approaches, and models of care. Essential elements of good geriatric primary care include the recognition of geriatric syndromes, evaluation of functional status, and the use of prognosis and patient goals in determining a realistic diagnostic and treatment plan. Innovative models of geriatric care delivery, including the GRACE, PACE, and

Hospital-at-Home programs, can improve geriatric care. Important elements of these care delivery models include improved access to a multidisciplinary team, periodic comprehensive geriatric assessment, medication reconciliation, and integration of palliative care into primary care. More widespread dissemination of these models would improve geriatric care nationwide. Clinicians providing care to the elderly without access to these models can improve care by using efficient screening tools for geriatric syndromes, recognizing frailty and its effect on prognosis, incorporating prognosis and patient preferences into medical decision-making, and using a multidisciplinary approach to care whenever possible.

REFERENCES

1. Centers for Disease Control and Prevention. Health, United States 2005. Available at: http://www.cdc.gov/nchs/data/hus/hus05.pdf. Accessed August 5, 2014.
2. Federal Interagency Forum on Aging-Related Statics. Older Americans 2010: key indicators of well-being. 2010. Available at: http://www.agingstats.gov/agingstatsdotnet/Main_Site/Data/2010_Documents/Docs/OA_2010.pdf. Accessed August 5, 2014.
3. Crippen DL. Disease management in Medicare: data analysis and benefit design issues. Washington, DC: Congressional Budget Office Testimony before the Special Committee on Aging, U.S. Senate; September 19, 2002.
4. Flacker J. What is a geriatric syndrome anyway? J Am Geriatr Soc 2003;51: 574–6.
5. Inouye SK, Studenski S, Tinetti ME, et al. Geriatric syndromes: clinical, research, and policy implications of a core geriatric concept. J Am Geriatr Soc 2007;55:780–91.
6. Creditor MC. Hazards of hospitalization of the elderly. Ann Intern Med 1993;118: 219–23.
7. Tinetti ME, Inouye SK, Gill TM, et al. Shared risk factors for falls, incontinence and functional dependence. Unifying the approach to geriatric syndromes. JAMA 1995;273:1348–53.
8. Inouye SK, Brown CJ, Tinetti ME. Medicare nonpayment, hospital falls, and unintended consequences. N Engl J Med 2009;360:2390–3.
9. Wayne PM, Walsh JN, Taylor-Piliae RE, et al. Effect of tai chi on cognitive performance in older adults: systematic review and meta-analysis. J Am Geriatr Soc 2014;62:25–39.
10. Wu G. Evaluation of the effectiveness of tai chi for improving balance and preventing falls in the older population—a review. J Am Geriatr Soc 2002;50:746–54.
11. Fried LP, Tangen CM, Walston J, et al. Frailty in older adults: evidence for a phenotype. J Gerontol A Biol Sci Med Sci 2001;56:M146–56.
12. Rodakowski J, Skidmore ER, Reynolds CF, et al. Can performance on daily activities discriminate between older adults with normal cognitive function and those with mild cognitive impairment? J Am Geriatr Soc 2014;62:1347–52.
13. Bogardus ST, Richardson E, Maciejewski PK, et al. Evaluation of a guided protocol for quality improvement in identifying common geriatric problems. J Am Geriatr Soc 2002;50:328–35.
14. Phelan EA, Genshaft S, Williams B, et al. How "geriatric" is care provided by fellowship-trained geriatricians compared to that of generalists? J Am Geriatr Soc 2008;56:1807–11.
15. American Geriatrics Society Expert Panel on the Care of Older Adults with Multimorbidity. Patient-centered care for older adults with multiple chronic conditions: a stepwise approach from the American Geriatrics Society: American Geriatrics

Society Expert Panel on the care of older adults with multimorbidity. J Am Geriatr Soc 2012;60:1957–68.

16. Gillespie LD, Robertson MC, Gillespie WJ, et al. Interventions for preventing falls in older people living in the community. Cochrane Database Syst Rev 2009;(2):CD007146.

17. Tinetti ME, Kumar C. The patient who falls. "It's always a trade-off." JAMA 2010; 303:258–66.

18. Panel on Prevention of Falls in Older Persons, American Geriatrics Society and British Geriatrics Society. Summary of the updated American Geriatrics Society/British Geriatrics Society clinical practice guideline for prevention of falls in older persons. J Am Geriatr Soc 2011;59:148–57.

19. Tinetti ME. Performance-oriented assessment of mobility problems in elderly patients. J Am Geriatr Soc 1986;34:119–26.

20. Guralnick JM, Simonsick EM, Ferrucci L, et al. A short physical performance battery assessing lower extremity function: association with self-reported disability and prediction of mortality and nursing home admission. J Gerontol A Biol Sci Med Sci 1994;49:M85–94.

21. Bogle Thorbahn LD, Newton RA. Use of the Berg balance test to predict falls in elderly persons. Phys Ther 1996;76:576–83.

22. Mathias S, Nayak US, Isaacs B. Balance in elderly patients: the "get-up and go" test. Arch Phys Med Rehabil 1986;34:119–26.

23. Duncan PW, Weiner DK, Chandler J, et al. Functional reach: a new clinical measure of balance. J Gerontol 1990;45:M192–7.

24. Moyer VA. Screening for cognitive impairment in older adults: U.S. Preventive Services Task Force recommendation statement. Ann Intern Med 2014;160:791–7.

25. Julayanont P, Brousseau M, Chertkow H, et al. Montreal cognitive assessment memory index score as a predictor of conversion from mild cognitive impairment to Alzheimer's disease. J Am Geriatr Soc 2012;62:679–84.

26. Nasreddine ZS, Phillips NA, Bedirian V, et al. The Montreal Cognitive Assessment, MoCA: a brief screening tool for mild cognitive impairment. J Am Geriatr Soc 2005;53:695–9.

27. Borson S, Scanlan J, Brush M, et al. The mini-cog: a cognitive 'vital signs' measure for dementia screening in multi-lingual elderly. Int J Geriatr Psychiatry 2000; 15:1021–7.

28. Hort J, O'Brien JT, Ganinotti G, et al. EFNS guidelines for the diagnosis and management of Alzheimer's disease. Eur J Neurol 2010;17:1236–48.

29. Resnick NM, Yalla SV. Management of urinary incontinence in the elderly. N Engl J Med 1985;313:800–5.

30. Khandelwal C, Kistler C. Diagnosis of urinary incontinence. Am Fam Physician 2013;87:543–50.

31. Brown JS, Bradley CS, Sebak LL, et al. The sensitivity and specificity of a simple test to distinguish between urge and stress urinary incontinence. Ann Intern Med 2006;144:715–23.

32. Barry MJ, Williford WO, Chang Y, et al. Benign prostatic hyperplasia specific health status measures in clinical research: how much change in the American Urological Association symptom index and the benign prostatic hyperplasia impact index is perceptible to patients? J Urol 1995;154:1770–4.

33. Coyne KS, Zyczynski T, Margolis MK, et al. Validation of an overactive bladder awareness tool for use in primary care settings. Adv Ther 2005;22:381–94.

34. Wilhelm-Leen ER, Hall YN, Tamura M, et al. Frailty and chronic kidney disease: the third National Health and Nutrition Evaluation Survey. Am J Med 2009;122:664–71.

35. Robinson TN, Wu DS, Pointer L, et al. Simple frailty score predicts postoperative complications across surgical specialties. Am J Surg 2013;206:544–50.
36. Ganapathi AM, Englum BR, Hanna JM, et al. Frailty and risk in proximal aortic surgery. J Thorac Cardiovasc Surg 2014;147:186–91.
37. Walker SR, Gill K, Macdonald K, et al. Association of frailty and physical function in patients with non-dialysis CKD: a systemic review. BMC Nephrol 2013;14:228.
38. Graham MM, Galbraith PD, O'Neill D, et al. Frailty and outcome in elderly patients with acute coronary syndrome. Can J Cardiol 2013;29:1610–5.
39. Mitniski AB, Mogliner AJ, Rockwood K. Accumulation of deficits as proxy measure of aging. ScientificWorldJournal 2001;1:323–36.
40. Armstrong JJ, Mitnitski A, Launer LJ, et al. Frailty in the Honolulu-Asia aging study: deficit accumulation in a male cohort followed to 90% mortality. J Gerontol A Biol Sci Med Sci 2015;70:125–31.
41. Malmstrom TK, Miller DK, Morley JE. A comparison of four frailty models. J Am Geriatr Soc 2014;62:721–6.
42. Abellan van Kan G, Rolland Y, Bergman H, et al. The I.A.N.A. task force on frailty assessment of older people in clinical practice. J Nutr Health Aging 2008;12: 29–37.
43. Ensrud KE, Ewing SK, Taylor BC, et al. Comparison of 2 frailty indexes for prediction of falls, disability, fractures and death in older women. Arch Intern Med 2008; 168:382–9.
44. Ravindrarajah R, Lee DM, Pye SR, et al. The ability of three different models of frailty to predict all-cause mortality: results from the European Male Aging Study (EMAS). Arch Gerontol Geriatr 2013;57:360–8.
45. Woo J, Leung J, Morley JE. Comparison of frailty indicators based on clinical phenotype and the multiple deficit approach in predicting mortality and physical limitation. J Am Geriatr Soc 2012;60:1478–86.
46. Tinetti ME, Fried TR, Boyd CM. Designing health care for the most common chronic condition–multimorbidity. JAMA 2012;307(23):2493–4.
47. Bielaszka-DuVernay C. The 'GRACE' model: in-home assessments lead to better care for dual eligibles. Health Aff (Millwood) 2011;30(3):431–4.
48. Komisar HL, Feder J. Transforming care for Medicare beneficiaries with chronic conditions and long-term care needs: coordinating care across all services, in National Health Policy Forum. The SCAN Foundation; 2011. Available at: www. TheSCANFoundation.org.
49. Master RJ, Eng C. Integrating acute and long-term care for high-cost populations. Health Aff (Millwood) 2001;20(6):161–72.
50. Hughes SL, Weaver FM, Giobbie-Hurder A, et al. Effectiveness of team-managed home-based primary care: a randomized multicenter trial. JAMA 2000;284(22): 2877–85.
51. Counsell SR, Frank K, Levine S, et al. Dissemination of GRACE care management to a managed care medical group. J Am Geriatr Soc 2011;59:S194–5.
52. Kinosian B, Meyer S, Yudin J, et al. Elder partnership for all-inclusive care (Elder-PAC): 5-year follow-up of integrating care for frail, community elders, linking home based primary care with an area agency on aging (AAA) as an independence at home (IAH) model. J Am Geriatr Soc 2010;58:S6.
53. Bodenheimer T, Berry-Millet R. Care management for people with complex health care needs. Synthesis Project: 19. Robert Wood Johnson Foundation; 2009. p. 2–40.
54. Coleman EA, Berenson RA. Lost in transition: challenges and opportunities for improving the quality of transitional care. Ann Intern Med 2004;141(7):533–6.

55. Coleman EA, Parry C, Chalmers S, et al. The care transitions intervention: results of a randomized controlled trial. Arch Intern Med 2006;166(17):1822–8.
56. Coleman EA, Rosenbek SA, Roman SP. Disseminating evidence-based care into practice. Popul Health Manag 2013;16(4):227–34.
57. Naylor MD. Transitional care for older adults: a cost-effective model. LDI Issue Brief 2004;9(6):1–4.
58. Naylor MD, Aiken LH, Kurtzman ET, et al. The care span: the importance of transitional care in achieving health reform. Health Aff (Millwood) 2011;30(4):746–54.
59. Boult C, Leff B, Boyd CM, et al. A matched-pair cluster-randomized trial of guided care for high-risk older patients. J Gen Intern Med 2013;28(5):612–21.
60. Meier DE, Thar W, Jordan A, et al. Integrating case management and palliative care. J Palliat Med 2004;7(1):119–34.
61. Sweeney L, Halpert A, Waranoff J. Patient-centered management of complex patients can reduce costs without shortening life. Am J Manag Care 2007;13(2): 84–92.
62. Wajnberg A, Ornstein K, Zhang M, et al. Symptom burden in chronically ill home-bound individuals. J Am Geriatr Soc 2013;61(1):126–31.
63. Eng C, Pedulla J, Eleazer GP, et al. Program of all-inclusive care for the elderly (PACE): an innovative model of integrated geriatric care and financing. J Am Geriatr Soc 1997;45:223–32.
64. Center for Health Systems Research and Analysis University of Wisconsin. Actuarial assessment of PACE enrollment characteristics in developing capitated payments. Available at: http://www.cms.gov/Research- Statistics-Data-and-Systems/Statistics-Trends-and-Reports/Reports/downloads/UofWi0307.pdf. Accessed August 4, 2014.
65. Counsell SR, Callahan CM, Clark DO, et al. Geriatric care management for low-income seniors: a randomized controlled trial. JAMA 2007;298:2623–33.
66. Counsell SR, Callahan CM, Tu W, et al. Cost analysis of the geriatric resources for assessment and care of elders care management intervention. J Am Geriatr Soc 2009;57:1420–6.
67. Cryer L, Shannon SB, Van Amsterdam M, et al. Costs for 'hospital at home' patients were 19 percent lower, with equal or better outcomes compared to similar inpatients. Health Aff (Millwood) 2012;31:1237–43.
68. Leff B, Burton L, Mader SL, et al. Hospital at Home: feasibility and outcomes of a program to provide hospital-level care at home for acutely ill older patients. Ann Intern Med 2005;143:798–808.
69. Naylor MD, Brooten D, Campbell R, et al. Comprehensive discharge planning and home follow-up of hospitalized elders: a randomized clinical trial. JAMA 1999;281:613–20.

Assessment and Management of Fall Risk in Primary Care Settings

 CrossMark

Elizabeth A. Phelan, MD, MS[a],*, Jane E. Mahoney, MD[b],
Jan C. Voit, PT[c], Judy A. Stevens, PhD[d]

KEYWORDS

- Accidental falls • Aged • Wounds and injuries • Primary prevention
- Secondary prevention • Risk assessment and management
- Preventive health services/organization and administration
- Community health services

KEY POINTS

- Falls are common and have adverse consequences, but are often preventable.
- Current guidelines specify that primary care providers should screen older adults for falls and risk for falling at least once a year by asking about falls and unsteadiness when walking.
- Multifactorial interventions that address many predisposing factors are appropriate for people at high risk and can decrease falls by approximately 25%.
- Three key risk factors (balance, medications, and home safety) should be addressed in everyone at high risk.
- Primary care providers should refer patients to clinical and community resources to address modifiable risk factors.

INTRODUCTION

Falls: Definition and Magnitude of the Problem

Falls occur more often with advancing age. Each year, approximately 30% to 40% of people aged 65 years and older who live in the community fall.[1] Roughly half of all falls

Disclaimer: The findings and conclusions in this report are those of the authors and do not necessarily represent the official position of the Centers for Disease Control and Prevention.
[a] Division of Gerontology and Geriatric Medicine, Harborview Medical Center, 325 9th Avenue, Box 359755, Seattle, WA 98104-2499, USA; [b] Division of Geriatrics and Gerontology, Department of Medicine, University of Wisconsin School of Medicine and Public Health, 310 North Midvale, Suite 205, Madison, WI 53705, USA; [c] Outpatient Physical and Hand Therapy Clinic, Harborview Medical Center, 908 Jefferson Street, Box 359920, Seattle, WA 98104-2499, USA; [d] National Center for Injury Prevention and Control, Centers for Disease Control and Prevention, 4770 Buford Highway, MS F-62, Atlanta, GA 30341, USA
* Corresponding author.
E-mail address: phelane@uw.edu

Med Clin N Am 99 (2015) 281–293
http://dx.doi.org/10.1016/j.mcna.2014.11.004
0025-7125/15/$ – see front matter © 2015 Elsevier Inc. All rights reserved.

result in an injury,[2] of which 10% are serious,[3] and injury rates increase with age.[4] The direct medical costs for falls total nearly $30 billion annually.[5]

Falls in the outpatient setting are usually defined as "coming to rest unintentionally on the ground or lower level, not due to an acute overwhelming event"[6] (eg, stroke, seizure, loss of consciousness) or external event to which any person would be susceptible.

Falls are a major threat to older adults' quality of life, often causing a decline in self-care ability and participation in physical and social activities. Fear of falling, which develops in 20% to 39% of people who fall, can lead to further limiting activity, independent of injury.[7]

Fall Risk Factors

Fall risk factors increase the likelihood that a person will fall. These risk factors can be categorized as extrinsic (external to the individual) and intrinsic (within-person) (**Fig. 1**). Intrinsic factors include several age-related physiologic changes, as summarized in **Table 1**.

Many falls result from interactions among multiple risk factors, and the risk of falling increases linearly with the number of risk factors.[1] However, even among community-dwelling people aged 75 years and older without risk factors, approximately 10% fall during any given year.[1] Therefore, all older adults should be recognized as being at some increased risk for falling.

Falls from Older Adults' Perspective

Older adults frequently think that falls are inevitable with aging[8] but underestimate their personal risk of falling.[9] Environmental and behavioral factors (eg, rushing, being distracted) are most often seen as causing falls; intrinsic (personal/health) factors are rarely recognized. Thus, primary care providers (PCPs) have a crucial role in helping patients understand the importance of intrinsic factors in causing falls.

Few older adults use proven fall prevention strategies such as balance exercises.[10] When asked what they are doing to prevent future falls, people commonly report being more careful.[11] However, there is no evidence that being more careful alone prevents falls.

Less than half of older adults who fall talk with their health care providers about it.[12] Therefore, guidelines specify that providers should ask all their patients aged 65 years

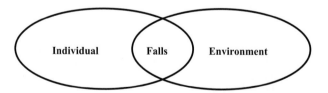

Age-related changes   Medications[a]
Cognitive deficits   Footwear[a]
Gait, strength, or balance deficits[a]   Assistive devices[a]
Sensory deficits[a]   Home/neighborhood features[a]
Chronic conditions   Alcohol/drugs[a]
Acute illnesses   Supports from caregivers[a]
Behaviors/choices[a]

Fig. 1. Falls result from an interaction between factors in the individual (intrinsic) and the environment (extrinsic). [a] Factors that may be modifiable with intervention.

Table 1
Aging-related physiologic changes in organ systems that affect fall risk

Organ System	Physiologic Change
Muscular system	Decreased muscle strength
Nervous System	
Balance	Increased postural sway Slowed righting reflexes
Gait	Decreased step height Decreased proprioception
Vision	Reduced papillary response to light variation Thickening and loss of elasticity of lens

and older about falls at least annually.[13] By evaluating patients for fall risk and encouraging them to adopt evidence-based prevention strategies, PCPs can help patients reduce their chances of falling and experiencing functional decline, injury, or death.

FALL RISK ASSESSMENT
Clinical Practice Guideline

A 2012 Cochrane Systematic Review reported that clinical assessment by a health care provider combined with individualized treatment of identified risk factors, referral if needed, and follow-up reduced the rate of falls by 24%.[14] Similarly, the US Preventive Services Task Force found that multifactorial clinical assessment and management, combined with follow-up, was effective in reducing falls.[15]

The American Geriatrics Society and British Geriatrics Society (AGS/BGS) have published a clinical practice guideline on fall risk screening, assessment, and management.[13] The AGS/BGS guideline[13] recommends screening all adults aged 65 years and older for fall risk annually. This screening consists of asking patients whether they have fallen 2 or more times in the past year or sought medical attention for a fall, or, if they have not fallen, whether they feel unsteady when walking. Patients who answer positively to any of these questions are at increased risk for falls and should receive further assessment. People who have fallen once without injury should have their balance and gait evaluated; those with gait or balance abnormalities should receive additional assessment. A history of 1 fall without injury and without gait or balance problems does not warrant further assessment beyond continued annual fall risk screening.[13]

A fall risk assessment is required as part of the Welcome to Medicare examination. PCPs can receive reimbursement for fall risk assessment through the Medicare Annual Wellness visit and incentive payments for assessing and managing fall risk through voluntary participation in the Physician Quality Reporting System.

Implementing Screening and Assessment

The US Centers for Disease Control and Prevention (CDC) has developed an algorithm that details each step of screening and assessment and guides interventions based on each individual's level of risk (**Fig. 2**).

This algorithm is part of a tool kit called STEADI (Stopping Elderly Accidents, Deaths, and Injuries).[16] Based on the AGS/BGS guideline[13] with input from practicing clinicians, STEADI was designed to help health care providers integrate falls assessment and management into their practice. The algorithm highlights that even

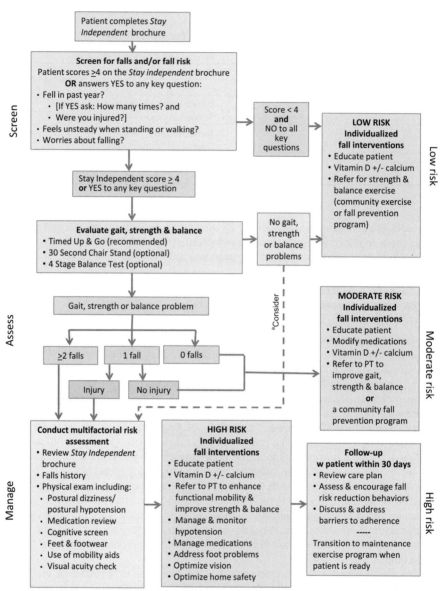

Fig. 2. STEADI (Stopping Elderly Accidents, Deaths, and Injuries) algorithm. [a] For patients who screen positive for falls but have no gait, strength, or balance problems, consider additional risk assessment (eg, medication review, cognitive screen, syncope). PT, physical therapist. (*From* Centers for Disease Control and Prevention. Algorithm for fall risk assessment & interventions. Available at: http://www.cdc.gov/homeandrecreationalsafety/pdf/steadi/algorithm_fall_risk_ assessment.pdf. Accessed November 11, 2014.)

individuals at low risk (no history of falls, no problems with gait or balance) can benefit from a primary prevention approach, namely education about fall risk factors, strength and balance exercises, and vitamin D supplementation.[15] The recommended dose of vitamin D for fall prevention is 1000 IU of cholecalciferol daily.[17]

Fall Risk Assessment

A risk assessment consists of a falls history, medication review, physical examination, and functional and environmental assessments.

The falls history

A falls history should include determining the number of falls in the past year as well as their circumstances, including any premonitory symptoms, location, activity, footwear, use of assistive device (if prescribed), use of glasses (if typically used), ability to get up after the fall, time of day, any injuries sustained, and any medical treatment received. Corroboration by a witness can be helpful in cases of recurrent, unexplained falls, because such falls may be caused by unrecognized syncope.[18] Documenting a falls history is one of the quality indicators for fall prevention and management.[19]

Medications and falls

A critical part of risk assessment is a medication review. Several classes of medications increase fall risk (**Table 2**). Psychoactive medications in particular are independent predictors of falls.[20] These medications tend to be sedating, alter the sensorium, and impair balance and gait. Other medications (eg, antihypertensives, nonsteroidal antiinflammatory drugs, diuretics) are more weakly associated with falls.[21]

A key strategy is to reduce the dose of any indicated medications that contribute to fall risk and to taper and stop any medications that are no longer indicated.[22] Nonpharmacologic approaches (eg, sleep hygiene measures for insomnia) are often a useful alternative.

Postural hypotension

Postural hypotension is defined as a reduction in systolic blood pressure of at least 20 mm Hg or in diastolic blood pressure of at least 10 mm Hg within 3 minutes of standing. Postural hypotension affects approximately 30% of community-dwelling older adults[23] and is a fall risk factor. Patients may experience lightheadedness, blurred vision, headache, fatigue, weakness, or syncope within 1 to several minutes of standing up, or they may be asymptomatic. In contrast, patients may experience postural lightheadedness without a measured blood pressure reduction; this should be considered equivalent to postural hypotension for fall risk. Postural hypotension can often be alleviated by reducing the dosage of blood pressure–lowering

Table 2 Medications that increase the risk of falls	
Medication Class	**Odds Ratio (95% CI)**
Psychoactive Medications	
Antidepressants	1.68 (1.47–1.91)
Antipsychotics	1.59 (1.37–1.83)
Sedative hypnotics	1.47 (1.35–1.62)
Benzodiazepines	1.57 (1.43–1.72)
Other Medications	
Antihypertensives	1.24 (1.01–1.50)
Nonsteroidal antiinflammatory drugs	1.21 (1.01–1.44)
Diuretics	1.07 (1.01–1.14)

Abbreviation: CI, confidence interval.
Data from Woolcott JC, Richardson KJ, Wiens MO, et al. Meta-analysis of the impact of 9 medication classes on falls in elderly persons. Arch Intern Med 2009;169:1957.

medications and/or stopping medications that have orthostatic hypotension as a side effect. Use of above-the-knee support hose and sleeping with the head of the bed elevated may also reduce postural reductions in blood pressure.

Fall-focused physical examination
The recommended elements of a fall-focused physical examination are shown in **Box 1**. An essential exam element is assessment of the patient's gait and balance. Three quick gait, strength, and balance tests are the Timed Up-and-Go (TUG), the 30-Second Chair Stand test, and the 4-Stage Balance test. These tests are described in the STEADI tool kit and shown in online instructional videos at: http://www.cdc.gov/homeandrecreationalsafety/Falls/steadi/index.html.

The TUG, a test of functional mobility, involves timing a person standing up from a chair with armrests (using their assistive device if they normally use one), walking 3 m (10 feet) at their usual pace, turning, returning to the chair, and sitting down. A TUG time greater than or equal to 12 seconds suggests high fall risk.[24]

The 30-Second Chair Stand test assesses lower extremity strength and balance. Being unable to stand up from a chair of knee height without using one's arms indicates increased fall risk.[20]

The 4-Stage Balance test assesses static balance by having the patient stand in 4 positions, each progressively more challenging. Positions include the parallel, semi-tandem, tandem, and single-leg stand.[25] Inability to perform a tandem stand (ie, heel of one shoe touching toe of the other) for 10 seconds predicts falls, and the inability to stand on 1 leg unassisted for 5 seconds predicts injurious falls.[26]

Cognitive testing is also an important part of the fall-related physical examination and may consist of a brief cognitive screen such as the Mini-Cog.[27] People with moderate to severe cognitive impairment are at high risk of falls.

Functional assessment
Assessing a patient's level of functioning is usually accomplished by asking standardized questions about difficulties with performing activities of daily living and instrumental

---

Box 1
Key elements of fall-focused physical examinations

Examination element

Orthostatic vital signs

Distance visual acuity

Cardiac examination (rate, rhythm, murmurs)

Gait and balance evaluation[a]

Musculoskeletal examination of back and lower extremities

Neurologic examination

  Cognitive screen

  Sensation

  Proprioception

  Muscle bulk, tone, strength, reflexes, and range of motion

  Higher neurologic function (cerebellar, motor cortex, basal ganglia)

[a] Recommended evaluations include the Timed Up-and-Go, 30-Second Chair Stand, and 4-Stage Balance tests.

activities of daily living. The risk of falling and the circumstances and location of falls vary by functional ability.[28] People who are healthier are more likely to fall on stairs, away from home, and during displacing activities (eg, bending over, reaching up), and are more likely to be seriously injured if they fall.[28] By contrast, people with functional limitations are more likely to fall at home during routine activities. Gauging functional ability can help determine the degree of fall and injury risk, indicate risk factors, and suggest interventions.

Laboratory tests and imaging

A comprehensive assessment may involve laboratory tests. These tests could include thyroid-stimulating hormone, vitamin B_{12} level, complete blood count, 25-hydroxy vitamin D level, and other laboratory tests if clinically indicated.[29]

A dual-energy x-ray absorptiometry scan should be done if bone mineral density has not been assessed. No other radiographic imaging study is routinely necessary. However, based on signs and symptoms, such as evidence of head injury or a new focal neurologic deficit, computed tomography or MRI of the brain may be indicated. An assessment for causes of syncope should be conducted only if there is strong suspicion, as in the case of recurrent, unexplained falls.

Environmental assessment

Environmental assessment, which is typically conducted by a trained health professional (eg, occupational therapist [OT]) on referral from the PCP, is intended to identify hazardous conditions within the home, such as obstacles in pathways or on stairs, unsupportive or ill-fitting footwear, unsuitable assistive devices, inadequate lighting, and slippery surfaces. It also identifies hazards outside the home, such as cracked pavement or sloped yards. Identifying and modifying environmental factors is an effective intervention as part of a comprehensive multifactorial approach to preventing falls.[13] It is also effective as a single intervention when delivered by an OT.[14] OTs consider behavioral factors that affect fall risk as well as adaptations that older adults can make to function safely in and around their homes.[30]

MANAGEMENT OF FALL RISK
Management Goals for Older Adults at Risk of Falls

Goals for fall risk management include (1) reduce the chances of falling, (2) reduce the risk of injury, (3) maintain the highest possible level of mobility, and (4) ensure ongoing follow-up.

Clinical Approach to Managing Fall Risk

Collaborate with patients and their caregivers to address fall risk factors

Providers should explore older adults' perceptions of the causes of their falls and willingness to make changes to reduce their risk of falling again. Approaches that facilitate behavior change include presenting the information that falls can be prevented, providing choices, personalizing options, and focusing strategies on enhancing quality of life (eg, maintaining independence).[8] The STEADI tool kit[16] includes guidance on talking about fall prevention with patients. There are examples of patients in various stages of readiness to make changes to reduce their fall risk, with possible provider responses for each stage.

Discuss the importance of strength and balance exercise

Exercise interventions that focus on improving strength and balance are the most effective single intervention for reducing falls and fall-related injuries.[14] Most older adults do not routinely practice these types of exercises.[31] Other forms of exercise (eg, stretching, walking) have not been shown to reduce falls.[32]

To be effective, exercise must (1) focus on improving balance, (2) be of moderate to high challenge and progress in difficulty, and (3) be practiced a minimum of 50 hours, which equates to 2 hours weekly for 25 weeks.[32] PCPs can educate patients about exercise that prevents falls and refer to appropriate resources (eg, physical therapists [PTs], community fall prevention programs) to initiate it. It is important to emphasize that the effects of exercise will not be apparent for several months, and that practice must be ongoing in order to maintain the benefits.

Evidence-based exercise programs may be either home based (eg, Otago Exercise Program[33]) or group classes offered in community settings (eg, tai chi[34]).

Prioritize interventions for modifiable risk factors

Because the risk of falling increases with the number of risk factors, risk can be reduced by modifying even a few contributing factors. Three key risk factors (balance, medications, and home safety) should be addressed in everyone at high risk.[35] In addition, if the PCP suspects that a cataract is affecting vision, it is beneficial to refer the patient for cataract extraction, assuming that the patient is a surgical candidate, because first eye cataract surgery decreases falls.[13,14]

In our experience, most high-risk patients are amenable to decreasing medication dosages and appreciate having their physician reduce the number of prescription medications. Most older adults are willing to consider balance training, especially if the instructions are not complicated and the exercises can be done at home.[36] A referral from a health care provider, particularly a physician, encourages follow-through with environmental assessment and modifications.[8]

Address fall injury risk

To reduce the chances of a fall injury, optimize bone health by recommending calcium and vitamin D supplementation and evaluating and treating osteoporosis.[15] Strengthening lower extremity muscles and teaching older adults how to get up from the ground after a fall may prevent a so-called long lie (remaining on the ground involuntarily because of inability to get up without help) with its associated medical complications.[37] High-risk patients should carry a cellular phone or wear a personal medical alert device to reduce the risk of a long lie in the event of a fall.

Involve relevant professional disciplines

Physical therapists PTs assess and treat balance, strength, and gait deficits. **Table 3** lists several tests that are typically done by PTs as part of a comprehensive gait and balance assessment.

PTs can design an exercise program to reduce fall risk that takes into consideration an individual's goals and functional abilities. The exercise program should be individually

Table 3 Tests for evaluation of gait and balance in people at risk of falls	
Test	**Purpose**
Dynamic Gait Index[43]	Gait with head turns, speed changes, and pivot turns; stepping over and around obstacles; chair-climbing
TUG Cognitive[24]	Gait with divided attention
Berg Balance Scale[44]	Balance with sitting, standing, transferring, reaching, and turning
Functional Reach[45]	Postural stability
Four Square Step Test[46]	Dynamic balance

Adapted from Refs.[24,43–46]

tailored to challenge balance. It may include static and dynamic activities as well as functional balance activities (eg, dual attention tasks, reaching and turning, weight shifting).

PTs work with older adults to improve their balance and mobility to the point where they can safely participate in a home or community exercise program. A PCP should initially refer a patient to a PT for a 3-month period of fall prevention exercise training. However, continued therapy beyond 3 months is frequently necessary before patients can successfully transition to a community program.[38]

With a referral from the PCP, PTs can determine whether patients require a mobility aid. PTs select and fit an assistive device and teach patients how to use it correctly.

Occupational therapists OTs assess the home environment and evaluate older adults' capacities (eg, vision, cognition) and deficits in relation to functioning safely within their homes. OTs elicit a falls history, individuals' beliefs about causes of falls, their understanding of environmental risks and perceived ability to negotiate those risks, and patterns of home use and community access.[30] OTs help older adults change their behavior to prevent falls; for example, by helping them create new routines during daily activities and identifying adaptive behaviors (eg, scanning ahead for hazards when walking). Like outpatient PT services, outpatient OT services are a covered Medicare Part B benefit. If patients meet Medicare's definition of homebound, they can receive home health services that can include a home safety evaluation by an OT under Medicare Part A.

Connect patients to evidence-based community fall prevention programs

Several effective fall prevention programs are becoming available in the community. For example, tai chi has been shown to reduce fall risk by 29%.[14] Some YMCAs are offering the tai chi program, Y-Moving for Better Balance. Stepping On, a 7-week workshop that teaches strength and balance exercises and behavior changes to prevent falls,[39] is also being disseminated (see https://wihealthyaging.org/stepping-on). Local public health departments and Area Agencies on Aging typically collaborate in community-level efforts to address falls.

Considerations for patients with dementia

Dementia impairs gait, balance, and hazard recognition. About half of community-dwelling older adults with dementia experience a fall every year.[1] Few randomized intervention studies have included people with dementia, and so current evidence is insufficient to recommend for or against a particular fall prevention intervention.[13] However, recent evidence suggests that the mobility and balance deficits seen in dementia may be improved through exercise.[40]

Working with the patient's caregiver becomes important in addressing fall risk in patients with dementia.[41] The caregiver can help by modifying the environment to improve safety and the way in which older adults with dementia perform mobility-related activities (eg, dressing, toileting, housekeeping) in and around the home. In some cases, it may be necessary to provide assistance with activities that the older adult can no longer safely perform. Their caregivers also may help older adults with dementia perform a set of basic exercises[42] or consistently use an assistive device. An evaluation by an OT is critical and should include observing how the patient performs mobility-related tasks in the home.

Offer ongoing monitoring and follow-up

Reducing falls using the clinical approach described herein requires ongoing monitoring by the providers.[35] Providers' active involvement can help ensure that patients act on recommendations. Providers can receive reimbursement for providing

Table 4
Resources for health care providers

Source	Item	Location
American Geriatrics Society	Clinical practice guideline on fall prevention	http://www.americangeriatrics.org/health_care_professionals/clinical_practice/clinical_guidelines_recommendations/prevention_of_falls_summary_of_recommendations
CDC	STEADI tool kit	www.cdc.gov/injury/steadi
Centers for Medicare and Medicaid Services	Welcome to Medicare (Initial Preventive Physical Examination) visit	www.cms.gov/Outreach-and-Education/Medicare-Learning-Network-MLN/MLNProducts/downloads/MPS_QRI_IPPE001a.pdf
Centers for Medicare and Medicaid Services	Annual Wellness visit	www.cms.gov/Outreach-and-Education/Medicare-Learning-Network-MLN/MLNProducts/Downloads/AWV_Chart_ICN905706.pdf
National Council on Aging	Fact sheets about Medicare coverage for fall-related clinical services	www.ncoa.org/improve-health/falls-prevention
National Institute on Aging	Go4Life exercise DVD and manual	http://go4life.nia.nih.gov

medically necessary fall-related services by using International Classification of Diseases, Tenth Revision, Clinical Modification (ICD-10-CM) code R29.6 for repeated falls.

For high-risk patients with multiple modifiable risk factors, it may be necessary to address each risk factor individually over time so as not to confuse or overwhelm the patient. These patients typically have multiple health issues and may see several specialists, all of whom make suggestions, adjust medications, and schedule the patient for follow-up visits.

A PCP managing a high-risk patient may complete assessments and recommend interventions over a 3-month period,[19] or longer if intercurrent health problems interfere. In this case, reassess the patient and recommend interventions at 4 to 6 months and as part of routine follow-up visits thereafter. Follow-up by other providers, (eg, nurse, PT, or OT) can augment the PCP's care.

Resources for clinical practice
Several resources can facilitate integrating fall prevention into practice (**Table 4**).

SUMMARY

Falls and their associated injuries are common and usually result from interactions among multiple fall risk factors, many of which may be modifiable. PCPs play a critical role in reducing fall risk factors among their older patients. Guidelines recommend annual screening to identify patients at increased risk of falling and comprehensive risk assessment and management of modifiable fall risk factors for high-risk patients. Regular exercise that improves strength and balance, along with vitamin D supplementation, can reduce falls and are appropriate prevention strategies even for low-risk patients. Understanding older adults' perspective and how to facilitate their involvement in fall prevention activities is critical to the success of provider efforts in this area.

REFERENCES

1. Tinetti ME, Speechley M, Ginter SF. Risk factors for falls among elderly persons living in the community. N Engl J Med 1988;319:1701–7.
2. King MB, Tinetti ME. Falls in community-dwelling older persons. J Am Geriatr Soc 1995;43:1146–54.
3. Tinetti ME, Doucette J, Claus E, et al. Risk factors for serious injury during falls by older persons in the community. J Am Geriatr Soc 1995;43:1214–21.
4. Schiller JS, Kramarow EA, Dey AN. Fall injury episodes among noninstitutional-ized older adults: United States, 2001-2003. Hyattsville, MD: National Center for Health Statistics Advance data from vital and health statistics 2007;392.
5. Stevens JA, Corso PS, Finkelstein EA, et al. The costs of fatal and non-fatal falls among older adults. Inj Prev 2006;12:290–5.
6. The prevention of falls in later life. A report of the Kellogg International Work Group on the Prevention of Falls by the Elderly. Dan Med Bull 1987;34:1–24.
7. Scheffer AC, Schuurmans MJ, van Dijk N, et al. Fear of falling: measurement strategy, prevalence, risk factors and consequences among older persons. Age Ageing 2008;37:19–24.
8. Bunn F, Dickinson A, Barnett-Page E, et al. A systematic review of older people's perceptions of facilitators and barriers to participation in falls-prevention interventions. Ageing Soc 2008;28:449–72.
9. Yardley L, Bishop FL, Beyer N, et al. Older people's views of falls-prevention interventions in six European countries. Gerontologist 2006;46:650–60.
10. Boyd R, Stevens JA. Falls and fear of falling: burden, beliefs and behaviours. Age Ageing 2009;38:423–8.
11. Calhoun R, Meischke H, Hammerback K, et al. Older adults' perceptions of clinical fall prevention programs: a qualitative study. J Aging Res 2011;2011:867341.
12. Stevens JA, Ballesteros MF, Mack KA, et al. Gender differences in seeking care for falls in the aged Medicare population. Am J Prev Med 2012;43:59–62.
13. Panel on Prevention of Falls in Older Persons. Summary of the Updated American Geriatrics Society/British Geriatrics Society clinical practice guideline for prevention of falls in older persons. J Am Geriatr Soc 2011;59:148–57.
14. Gillespie LD, Robertson MC, Gillespie WJ, et al. Interventions for preventing falls in older people living in the community. Cochrane Database Syst Rev 2012;(9):CD007146.
15. Moyer VA. Prevention of falls in community-dwelling older adults: U.S. Preventive Services Task Force recommendation statement. Ann Intern Med 2012;157:197–204.
16. Stevens JA, Phelan EA. Development of STEADI: a fall prevention resource for health care providers. Health Promot Pract 2013;14:706–14.
17. American Geriatrics Society Workgroup on Vitamin D Supplementation for Older Adults. Recommendations abstracted from the American Geriatrics Society Consensus Statement on vitamin D for Prevention of Falls and Their Consequences. J Am Geriatr Soc 2014;62:147–52.
18. Richardson DA, Bexton RS, Shaw FE, et al. Prevalence of cardioinhibitory carotid sinus hypersensitivity in patients 50 years or over presenting to the accident and emergency department with "unexplained" or "recurrent" falls. Pacing Clin Electrophysiol 1997;20:820–3.
19. Chang JT, Ganz DA. Quality indicators for falls and mobility problems in vulnerable elders. J Am Geriatr Soc 2007;55(Suppl 2):S327–34.

20. Ganz DA, Bao Y, Shekelle PG, et al. Will my patient fall? JAMA 2007;297:77–86.
21. Woolcott JC, Richardson KJ, Wiens MO, et al. Meta-analysis of the impact of 9 medication classes on falls in elderly persons. Arch Intern Med 2009;169: 1952–60.
22. Tinetti ME, Baker DI, McAvay G, et al. A multifactorial intervention to reduce the risk of falling among elderly people living in the community. N Engl J Med 1994; 331:821–7.
23. Poon IO, Braun U. High prevalence of orthostatic hypotension and its correlation with potentially causative medications among elderly veterans. J Clin Pharm Ther 2005;30:173–8.
24. Shumway-Cook A, Brauer S, Woollacott M. Predicting the probability for falls in community-dwelling older adults using the Timed Up & Go Test. Phys Ther 2000;80:896–903.
25. Rossiter-Fornoff JE, Wolf SL, Wolfson LI, et al. A cross-sectional validation study of the FICSIT common data base static balance measures. Frailty and Injuries: Cooperative Studies of Intervention Techniques. J Gerontol A Biol Sci Med Sci 1995;50:M291–7.
26. Vellas BJ, Wayne SJ, Romero L, et al. One-leg balance is an important predictor of injurious falls in older persons. J Am Geriatr Soc 1997;45:735–8.
27. Borson S, Scanlan JM, Chen P, et al. The Mini-Cog as a screen for dementia: validation in a population-based sample. J Am Geriatr Soc 2003;51:1451–4.
28. Speechley M, Tinetti M. Falls and injuries in frail and vigorous community elderly persons. J Am Geriatr Soc 1991;39:46–52.
29. Tinetti ME. Preventing falls in elderly persons. N Engl J Med 2003;348:42–9.
30. Peterson EW, Clemson L. Understanding the role of occupational therapy in fall prevention for community-dwelling older adults. OT Practice 2008;13:CE1–8.
31. Merom D, Pye V, Macniven R, et al. Prevalence and correlates of participation in fall prevention exercise/physical activity by older adults. Prev Med 2012;55: 613–7.
32. Sherrington C, Whitney JC, Lord SR, et al. Effective exercise for the prevention of falls: a systematic review and meta-analysis. J Am Geriatr Soc 2008;56: 2234–43.
33. Campbell AJ, Robertson MC, Gardner MM, et al. Randomised controlled trial of a general practice programme of home based exercise to prevent falls in elderly women. BMJ 1997;315:1065–9.
34. Li F, Harmer P, Fisher KJ, et al. Tai Chi and fall reductions in older adults: a randomized controlled trial. J Gerontol A Biol Sci Med Sci 2005;60:187–94.
35. Tinetti ME, Kumar C. The patient who falls: "It's always a trade-off". JAMA 2010; 303:258–66.
36. Yardley L, Kirby S, Ben-Shlomo Y, et al. How likely are older people to take up different falls prevention activities? Prev Med 2008;47:554–8.
37. Mallinson WJ, Green MF. Covert muscle injury in aged patients admitted to hospital following falls. Age Ageing 1985;14:174–8.
38. Shubert TE. Evidence-based exercise prescription for balance and falls prevention: a current review of the literature. J Geriatr Phys Ther 2011;34:100–8.
39. Clemson L, Cumming RG, Kendig H, et al. The effectiveness of a community-based program for reducing the incidence of falls in the elderly: a randomized trial. J Am Geriatr Soc 2004;52:1487–94.
40. Suttanon P, Hill K, Said C. Can balance exercise programme improve balance and related physical performance measures in people with dementia? A systematic review. Eur Rev Aging Phys Act 2010;7:13–25.

41. Mahoney JE, Shea TA, Przybelski R, et al. Kenosha County Falls Prevention Study: a randomized, controlled trial of an intermediate-intensity, community-based multifactorial falls intervention. J Am Geriatr Soc 2007;55:489–98.
42. Logsdon RG, McCurry SM, Teri L. A home health care approach to exercise for persons with Alzheimer's disease. Care Manag J 2005;6:90–7.
43. VanSwearingen JM, Paschal KA, Bonino P, et al. Assessing recurrent fall risk of community-dwelling, frail older veterans using specific tests of mobility and the physical performance test of function. J Gerontol A Biol Sci Med Sci 1998;53:M457–64.
44. Berg KO, Wood-Dauphinee SL, Williams JI, et al. Measuring balance in the elderly: validation of an instrument. Can J Public Health 1992;83(Suppl 2):S7–11.
45. Duncan PW, Weiner DK, Chandler J, et al. Functional reach: a new clinical measure of balance. J Gerontol 1990;45:M192–7.
46. Dite W, Temple VA. A clinical test of stepping and change of direction to identify multiple falling older adults. Arch Phys Med Rehabil 2002;83:1566–71.

Appropriate Prescribing and Important Drug Interactions in Older Adults

Jeffrey Wallace, MD, MPH[a],*, Douglas S. Paauw, MD, MACP[b]

KEYWORDS

- Elderly • Polypharmacy • Drug interactions • Adverse drug events
- Potentially inappropriate medications • Adherence

KEY POINTS

- Polypharmacy, the use of 5 or more medications, is common in older adults.
- Polypharmacy is associated with increased rates of adverse drug events, use of potentially inappropriate medications, and increased drug interactions.
- Clinicians need to be aware of drug-drug and drug-disease interactions that are common and important.
- Tools and approaches to reducing polypharmacy can enhance the care and health outcomes of older adults.

INTRODUCTION

Adults 65 years of age and older represent 14% of the US population, but take 30% of prescription medications and 50% of over-the-counter medications.[1] Most adverse drug events occur in older adults, a fact that is attributable to their greater use of medications, increased vulnerability from underlying medical conditions, and age-related physiologic changes (**Box 1**).[2] The elderly also often suffer from suboptimal medication prescribing that ranges from underuse to overuse to misuse of medications. This article provides clinicians with approaches to optimize medication management in older adults with a focus on reducing polypharmacy and complications related to polypharmacy, medication adherence, use of potentially inappropriate medications, adverse drug reactions, and clinically important drug interactions in older adults.

[a] Division of Geriatric Medicine, Department of Internal Medicine, University of Colorado School of Medicine, 12631 East 17th Avenue, B-179, Aurora, CO 80045, USA; [b] Division of General Internal Medicine, Department of Medicine, University of Washington, 4245 Roosevelt way NE, #MC354760, Seattle, WA 98105, USA
* Corresponding author.
E-mail address: jeff.wallace@ucdenver.edu

Med Clin N Am 99 (2015) 295–310
http://dx.doi.org/10.1016/j.mcna.2014.11.005
0025-7125/15/$ – see front matter © 2015 Elsevier Inc. All rights reserved.

medical.theclinics.com

> **Box 1**
> **Age-related changes that increase susceptibility to adverse drug effects**
>
> *Pharmacodynamic changes: altered sensitivity to medications (very few)*
>
> Increased sensitivity
>
> • Warfarin, opiates
>
> Decreased sensitivity
>
> • β-agonists
>
> *Pharmacokinetic changes: alterations in factors that affect drug concentration*
>
> **Absorption:** minimal clinical relevance (ie, if med is swallowed it generally will be absorbed)
>
> **Distribution:** significant clinical relevance but not readily predictable
>
> • Increased fat mass increases volume distribution and half-life of lipophilic medications
>
> • Decreased total body water results in decreased volume of distribution and increased concentration of water-soluble drugs
>
> • Decreased fat-free mass/plasma protein leads to higher percentage of unbound (active) drug
>
> **Hepatic metabolism:** some clinical relevance but not consistently predictable
>
> • Decreased first-pass metabolism leads to increased concentration of drugs that typically have high levels of first-pass metabolism (ie, hepatic clearance before reaching systemic circulation)
>
> • Diazepam, propranolol, lidocaine
>
> **Renal clearance:** significant impact and readily predictable
>
> • Increased concentration of renally cleared drugs
>
> • Serum creatinine alone does *not* provide adequate information to guide dosing
>
> • Use Cockcroft-Gault (CG)[a] to estimate glomerular filtration rate (eGFR)
>
>   ○ More conservative that other calculations (eg, modification of diet in renal disease [MDRD]), less likely to overestimate eGFR, especially in frail older adults
>
>   ○ Drug company renal dose recommendations are based on CG
>
> [a] CG = $[(140 - age) \times wt (kg)] \times 0.85$ if female/($72 \times$ serum creatinine).

POLYPHARMACY

Polypharmacy, defined as taking 5 or more medications a day, is common in older adults.[3,4] One national survey found that more than 50% of female Medicare beneficiaries took 5 or more medications daily, with 12% taking 10 or more medications a day.[5] Although use of 5 or more medications often appears to be mandated by evidence-based care guidelines, evidence is generally lacking for applying such guidelines to older patients with multiple medical conditions. Conversely, evidence indicates that the use of more medications is associated with increased medication side effects and adverse health events, and these risks increase in a nonlinear fashion as number of drugs increases to 5 or more (**Fig. 1**). One study found that when compared with persons taking 4 or fewer medications, the risk of an adverse drug reaction nearly doubled (odds ratio [OR] 1.9, 95% confidence interval [CI] 1.35–2.68) for persons taking 5 to 7 medications, and quadrupled (OR 4.07, 95% CI 2.93–5.65) for those taking 8 or more medications.[4] Although not always inappropriate, the use of 5 or more medications is associated with higher rates of unwanted health outcomes (**Box 2**).[4,6] These and other issues related to polypharmacy are outlined in this section.

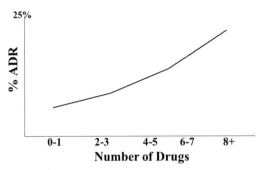

Fig. 1. Association between polypharmacy and adverse drug reactions (ADR). (*Data from* Onder G, Petrovic M, Tangiisuran B, et al. Development and validation of a score to assess risk of adverse drug reactions among in-hospital patients 65 years or older: the GerontoNet ADR risk score. Arch Intern Med 2010;170(13):1142.)

MULTIMORBIDITY AND GUIDELINE IMPLICATIONS

Twenty percent of Medicare beneficiaries have 5 or more chronic conditions. Higher levels of multimorbidity (presence of multiple chronic diseases) are associated with an increased prevalence of polypharmacy, owing in part to guidelines that call for pharmacologic management of each of the multiple medical conditions that an older adult may have.[7] However, the coexistence of multiple medical conditions and poly-pharmacy increases the potential for older adults to have more medication-related complications, ranging from difficulties managing their medications to increased rates of adverse medication effects.[8,9] Few studies have enrolled significant numbers of this vulnerable population, older adults with multimorbidity and polypharmacy, to help discern if potential benefits of increased medication use outweighs potential risks.[10] Clinicians are thus faced with an evidence/data gap in addressing medication use in older frail patients. Although this may feel disconcerting in this era of evidence-based care, it increases opportunities and impetus for clinicians to carefully evaluate the risk-benefit of each medication and work collaboratively with patients to ensure that medication regimens fit patient preferences and goals of care.

USE OF HIGH-RISK AND POTENTIALLY INAPPROPRIATE MEDICATIONS

It is estimated that 20% to 65 % of older adults take potentially inappropriate medications.[11] Clinicians should be familiar with well-known comprehensive reviews that

Box 2
Problems associated with polypharmacy
Adverse drug reactions
Drug-drug interactions
Drug-disease interactions
Higher risk for use of potentially inappropriate medications
Decreased adherence
Increased risk for medication errors
Increased cost
Increased morbidity and mortality

provide lists of medications that should be used cautiously or not at all in older adults, such as the Beers Criteria[12] and the annually updated list of high-risk medications in older adults published by The Healthcare Effectiveness Data and Information Set.[13] However, two-thirds of adverse drug effects that result in emergency room visits and hospitalizations in older adults are not due to potentially inappropriate medications, but rather to the following 4 medications: warfarin and antiplatelet agents (due to bleeding), and insulin and sulfonylurea agents (due to hypoglycemia).[14] When prescribing these 4 agents with high potential for serious adverse events, clinicians should intermittently assess if their continued use is providing health benefits that outweigh potential risks. It is also important to recognize that when aspirin is being used for cardioprotection in patients with *stable* coronary artery disease, it may be safely discontinued when such patients develop an indication for ongoing anticoagulation with warfarin. For example, if a patient with previous myocardial infarction taking daily aspirin develops atrial fibrillation or has a new thromboembolic event that leads to initiation of warfarin, aspirin should be discontinued because warfarin is cardioprotective. Continuing both warfarin and aspirin doubles the risk of bleeding without conferring additional cardioprotection relative to warfarin alone.[15,16] A selected list of frequently problematic medications that should be used with caution or not at all in older adults is presented in **Table 1**.

MEDICATION ADHERENCE AND ERRORS

Adherence to medication regimens is often problematic in patients of all ages.[17] Nonadherence rates often approach 50% after 1 year, even for such seemingly important medications as aspirin, statins, and β-blockers following a myocardial infarction.[18] Although there are many potential reasons for poor compliance with medications that should be explored with patients (**Table 2**), several studies indicate that

Table 1
Selected medications that should be avoided in older adults

Medication	Potential Harm/Concern
Muscle relaxants (eg, cyclobenzaprine, methocarbamol)	Sedating, anticholinergic, increased fall and fracture risk, uncertain efficacy.
Megestrol acetate	Not well proven and minimal effect on weight gain in older adults, lag time of several weeks to months for possible beneficial effect, increased risk of thrombotic events, increased mortality risk.
Iron more than once daily	Increased gastrointestinal side effects (eg, nausea, constipation) usually outweigh small marginal gains in iron absorbed when daily dose increased to twice a day (and even smaller marginal gains when increase twice-daily dose to 3 times a day).
Chronic daily nonsteroidal anti-inflammatory drug use	Gastrointestinal bleed, renal insufficiency, fluid retention, blood pressure elevation. Short-term use for acute injury/acute pain may be appropriate.
Chronic benzodiazepine use	Fall risk, confusion, dependency/withdrawal. Better/safer agents available for sleep and anxiety, including nonpharmacological.
First-generation antihistamines (eg, diphenhydramine)	Sedating, anticholinergic effects: confusion, dry mouth, dry eyes, constipation, urinary retention.

Table 2
Potential reasons for poor compliance with medications

Issue	Approaches to Improve Adherence
High number of drugs and regimen complexity	Limit number of medications, ideally to <5; simplify regimens using once-daily dosing whenever possible.
Inadequate patient understanding	Include drug indication on prescription: if you write it on rx, it will be on the bottle! Whenever initiating new drug explain rationale and anticipated duration of therapy.
Prescription not congruent with patient goals, cost barriers	Elicit nonadherence with nonjudgmental questions[19] (eg, "I know it must be difficult to take all your medications regularly. How often do you miss taking them?") Explore reasons if nonadherence is identified.
Memory problems, poor organization	Medication organizers, blister packs, electronic dispensing devices, cues/calls, monitoring, drug administration.
Difficulty taking (eg, vision or dexterity problems, pill dysphagia)	Order easy-to-remove bottle caps, larger-font labeling, magnifying glass, spacer for inhalers. For swallowing difficulties, explore if smaller tablets, solutabs, or liquid version substitutes are available.

medication number (polypharmacy) and regimen complexity are key factors.[19–21] This adds to the impetus to limit both the number of medications prescribed and to simplify the regimen (eg, daily vs twice or 3 times daily dosing) whenever possible. Polypharmacy increases the likelihood of patient errors when taking medications, and prescribing errors by providers are also more likely to occur when a greater total number of drugs is prescribed.[11] Adherence may be improved and medication errors reduced by limiting number of prescribers, using a single pharmacy, seeing patients more often, and synchronizing medication refills.

IMPORTANT DRUG INTERACTIONS IN THE ELDERLY
Overview

In addition to polypharmacy, the problem of drug interactions is heightened in older patients because of age-related decreases in metabolism and clearance of drugs, as well as increased vulnerability to drug interactions due to underlying comorbid conditions. There are thousands of potential drug interactions that can occur in elderly patients, and sorting out which are minor and which can be critically important is daunting. This section highlights a few of the most common, dangerous, and problematic drug interactions in older adults.

Warfarin Interactions

Many elderly patients take warfarin chronically to reduce stroke risk from atrial fibrillation or to decrease risk of recurrent thromboembolic disease or thrombotic risk due to mechanical heart valves. The newer anticoagulants (direct thrombin inhibitors and Xa inhibitors) have far fewer problems with drug interactions than warfarin, but have potential shortcomings of not being reversible in the event of bleeding and posing a greater risk for lack of efficacy with missed doses (see the article by Rondina and colleagues elsewhere in this issue). Several drugs can interact with warfarin and reduce the effectiveness of the drug, increasing thrombotic risk. The agents that decrease the effectiveness of warfarin are antiseizure drugs, such as phenytoin, carbamazepine, and phenobarbital. Rifampin also increases the metabolism of warfarin. Binding agents, such as cholestyramine, can decrease absorption of warfarin, which reduces anticoagulant effect.

Much more common are drugs that decrease warfarin metabolism and can cause excessive anticoagulation. Many drugs have small effects on warfarin metabolism, but when given with other drugs that have bigger effects, the cumulative effect can be great. Good examples of drugs with slight effect on metabolism that can be additive are the drugs simvastatin and omeprazole. Trimethoprim-sulfamethoxazole is the most common drug to cause a severe elevation in international normalized ratio (INR) in patients taking warfarin. The effect can occur as early as 2 days after starting trimethoprim-sulfa, and the effect peaks at about 7 days. In a study of patients receiving antibiotics while taking warfarin, the average increase in INR was 1.76 for the patients taking trimethoprim-sulfa.[22] In this same study, quinolone use increased the INR by 0.85. Excessive anticoagulation due to quinolone-warfarin interaction is very much influenced by whether the patient is taking multiple other medications with minor interactions with warfarin. Azithromycin has a smaller interaction with warfarin, with the average increase in INR of 0.51. See **Box 3** for a list of common drugs with significant interactions with warfarin.

Acetaminophen is frequently used to treat pain in elderly patients. It is usually recommended to elderly patients as the first-line pain reliever of choice because it does not pose risk of gastrointestinal bleeding, cardiovascular risk, or renal toxicity. In patients taking warfarin, it is also recommended because it does not have an antiplatelet effect. However, acetaminophen does have an important interaction with warfarin. Hylek and colleagues[23] conducted a case-control study and found that patients on warfarin ingesting 9100 mg or more of acetaminophen a week for more than 1 week had a 10-fold increased risk of having an INR greater than 6. Mahe and colleagues[24]

Box 3
Common drugs that can increase international normalized ratio in patients taking warfarin

Greatest effect

Trimethoprim-sulfamethoxazole

Erythromycin

Metronidazole

Fluconazole

Itraconazole

Ketoconazole

Amiodarone

Important effect

Acetaminophen

Quinolones

Omeprazole

Esomeprazole

Azithromycin

conducted a placebo-controlled, double-blind, crossover trial to look at the effect of acetaminophen on anticoagulation with warfarin. The mean age of patients in this study was 62. Patients in the study received 4 g acetaminophen a day or placebo while they were taking a stable warfarin dose, then crossed over. The mean maximum INR when patients received acetaminophen was 3.45 compared with 2.66 when receiving placebo. Zhang and colleagues[25] studied the effect of 2 or 3 g acetaminophen daily on patients taking warfarin. Forty-five patients on stable warfarin therapy were randomized to acetaminophen 2 or 3 g daily or placebo. The mean increase in INR was 0.70 for those receiving 2 g acetaminophen a day and 0.67 for those receiving 3 g a day. The study population had an average age of 55 in the 2-g warfarin group, 47 in the 3-g warfarin group. Patients who use acetaminophen regularly and are taking warfarin should be closely monitored by checking an INR within the first week of starting daily dosing of acetaminophen. The prospective studies looking at the effect of acetaminophen on anticoagulation have not looked at elderly populations, so the increase in INR may even be greater in elderly patients than what has been reported in the literature.

Proton Pump Inhibitors

Many elderly patients are on chronic proton pump inhibitors (PPIs). PPIs can reduce the absorption of several medications and supplements, including thyroid hormone.[26] Absorption of the antifungal agents itraconazole and ketoconazole are markedly affected by high gastric pH. Neither of these medications should be given to patients taking PPIs unless the PPI is stopped. Dipyridamole is another medication commonly used in the elderly that can have absorption diminished by PPI use.[27] The absorption of nifedipine, digoxin, and alendronate is increased in the setting of increased gastric pH.[28] The effect is modest for digoxin and nifedipine, but bioavailability is double when alendronate is given in the setting of a high gastric pH.[28]

Clopidogrel is frequently prescribed to elderly patients after coronary stents are placed or for stroke prevention. The PPIs omeprazole and esomeprazole have an effect on CYP2C19-mediated conversion of clopidogrel to its active metabolite, and may reduce the effect of clopidogrel on platelet reactivity. However, recent studies have not shown an increase in poor cardiovascular outcomes because of this potential drug interaction in large populations.[29,30] One possible explanation for the lack of poor outcomes related to this interaction is that CYP2C19 genotype groups have different risk for clinically important susceptibility to this drug interaction.[31] Given this uncertainty, the Food and Drug Administration (FDA) has recently recommended labeling changes that the PPIs omeprazole and esomeprazole should be avoided in patients taking clopidogrel.[32]

Elderly patients are at much higher risk for osteoporosis than the younger population. PPI use can decrease the absorption of both calcium and magnesium.[33] Multiple studies, including meta-analyses, have shown increased fracture risk in PPI users.[34,35] This problem seems to be dose-related. The FDA has issued warnings on the increased fracture risk with PPIs.[36] PPIs also reduce Vitamin B12 absorption, increasing the risk of Vitamin B12 deficiency.[37]

Calcium Channel Blockers

Calcium channel blockers are commonly prescribed for elderly patients to treat hypertension and to help with rate control in patients with atrial fibrillation. Many elderly patients also are taking statins, and there is an important interaction between verapamil or diltiazem and the statins simvastatin, lovastatin, and to a lesser degree atorvastatin. The interaction between simvastatin and verapamil or diltiazem can raise the area under the curve (AUC) for simvastatin by twofold to fourfold.[38] It is recommended that no more than 10 mg of simvastatin be prescribed if diltiazem or verapamil are co-prescribed. Amlodipine has a more modest, but appreciable interaction with simvastatin and lovastatin, raising the AUC 1.5 to 1.7. The AUC is raised by 50% with the use of diltiazem with atorvastatin.[38] Fluvastatin, pravastatin, and rosuvastatin metabolism are not significantly altered by coadministration of a calcium channel blocker, and are good options for patients who need to take a statin and a calcium channel blocker.

Macrolide antibiotics, especially clarithromycin and erythromycin, have a major impact on the metabolism of calcium channel blockers. Clarithromycin and erythromycin are potent inhibitors of the cytochrome P450 3A4 enzyme that metabolizes calcium channel blockers. In a recent retrospective study, co-prescribing of clarithromycin or erythromycin and calcium channel blockers (most commonly amlodipine) was associated with an increased risk of hospitalization for acute renal failure.[39] This problem was not seen with co-prescribing of azithromycin. The mechanism for the acute renal failure is likely due to hypotension. Another study showed increased rates of hospitalization for hypotension in elderly patients receiving calcium channel blockers co-prescribed with clarithromycin or erythromycin.[40] There was no increased rate of hospitalizations for hypotension in patients prescribed azithromycin and calcium channel blockers. Patients who are on a calcium channel blocker should not receive clarithromycin or erythromycin. Azithromycin is a safe, appropriate alternative.

IMPORTANT DRUG SIDE EFFECTS UNIQUE TO THE ELDERLY
Selective Serotonin Reuptake Inhibitors

Elderly patients are more likely to develop hyponatremia with the use of selective serotonin reuptake inhibitors (SSRIs). The hyponatremia can be severe, and has been reported with multiple drugs in this class.[41] The serotonin-norepinephrine reuptake inhibitors (SNRIs) duloxetine and venlafaxine also have been associated with the development of hyponatremia in the elderly.[42,43] Cases have been reported in which patients who developed hyponatremia on an SSRI redeveloped hyponatremia when switched to an SNRI.[44] Risk factors for the development of SSRI-induced hyponatremia are preexisting lower baseline serum sodium level, advanced age, female sex, low body mass, and use of a diuretic.[41]

Use of selective serotonin uptake inhibitors also has been shown to increase the risk of upper gastrointestinal bleeding.[45] The risk of gastrointestinal bleeding is further increased by nonsteroidal anti-inflammatory drug (NSAID) use, with the risk being significantly higher than the risk posed by NSAIDs alone.[46] The increase in risk occurs early in the course of SSRI use.[47] Elderly patients are at higher risk for gastrointestinal bleeding due to NSAIDS, and appear to be at higher risk with SSRIs, with the combination putting them at significant risk for upper gastrointestinal bleeding.[48] Elderly patients who receive daily NSAID treatment should receive antiulcer therapy, and this is of utmost importance in patients who are also receiving SSRI treatment, as the already high bleeding risk due to NSAIDs is much higher with the coadministration of SSRIs.

Quinolones

Fluoroquinolones are frequently prescribed for the treatment of urinary tract infections and pneumonias in elderly patients. There are several side effects of fluoroquinolones that are important and more frequent in elderly patients. Renal function declines with age, and renal excretion is important for the quinolones, especially for levofloxacin, in which almost 90% is excreted unchanged in the urine, but still important for ciprofloxacin, with 50% excreted unchanged in the urine. Renal dose adjustments are important to avoid central nervous system (CNS) side effects. The CNS side effects include anxiety, restlessness, insomnia, hallucinations, psychosis, and seizures.[49] The CNS symptoms related to quinolones are often mistaken for signs of delirium due to infection or concern for CNS infection. Elderly patients with pronounced atherosclerotic disease of the CNS or with a seizure disorder are at higher risk for CNS toxicity from quinolones.

Tendonitis and tendon rupture are well-known side effects of quinolones and a black box warning exists to alert physicians of this important side effect. Elderly patients are at higher risk for tendonitis and tendon rupture.[50] Corticosteroid use also markedly increases the risk of tendonitis and rupture. Tendon rupture can occur any time after starting quinolones and for several months after stopping the drug.

Peripheral neuropathy is a common problem in elderly patients due to aging, as well as chronic diabetes, alcoholism, and many rarer causes. Quinolones have been implicated as a cause of peripheral neuropathy. The FDA issued a warning in August 2013 about the association of quinolone use and the acute development of neuropathy. The neuropathy can begin within days of receiving intravenous or oral quinolones.[51]

Trimethoprim-Sulfamethoxazole

There has been a marked increase in usage of trimethoprim-sulfamethoxazole in the past few years because of the emergence of community-acquired methicillin-resistant *Staphylococcus aureus*. More elderly patients are being treated with this medication, and the potential for problems with this drug have grown. Elderly patients are at risk for the development of hyperkalemia with trimethoprim-sulfamethoxazole. Antoniou and colleagues[52] studied hyperkalemia in elderly patients admitted to the hospital taking angiotensin-converting enzyme inhibitors (ACEIs) or angiotensin receptor blockers (ARBs), who had started an antibiotic in the previous 14 days. There was a relative risk of 6.7 (CI 4.5–10) for hyperkalemia-associated hospitalization in patients taking trimethoprim-sulfamethoxazole, with no increased risk in patients receiving other antibiotics (amoxicillin, ciprofloxacin, norfloxacin, and nitrofurantoin). The average age of the patients in this study was 82. Witt and colleagues[53] studied the effect of standard-dose trimethoprim-sulfamethoxazole on serum potassium in elderly men at a Department of Veterans Affairs hospital. In the study, all patients on drugs that could increase potassium (ACEIs, ARBs, potassium-sparing diuretics, NSAIDs, and β-blockers) or had chronic renal insufficiency were excluded. They compared the potassium levels of patients who received trimethoprim-sulfamethoxazole compared with those who received other antibiotics (amoxicillin and cephradine). The serum potassium concentration in the group that received trimethoprim-sulfamethoxazole was 4.22 ± 0.40 mmol/L and increased by 0.31 ± 0.38 mmol/L at the end of therapy. There was no change in the serum potassium levels in patients who received other antibiotics. It is important to be cautious with the use of trimethoprim-sulfamethoxazole in the elderly, especially those with renal insufficiency and on drugs that can cause hyperkalemia.

REDUCING POLYPHARMACY
Overview

Many thoughtful approaches have been suggested, and tools are available, to help clinicians improve prescribing in older adults.[6,54] The STOPP/START instrument is one example of a tool to help clinicians identify both overprescribing and underprescribing.[55] The latter refers to situations in which an older patient is not receiving a medication that is clearly indicated (eg, a relatively healthy 75-year-old woman with hypertension, mild proteinuria, and diabetes who is not on an ACEI). Application of the STOPP/START instrument to 400 older inpatients accompanied by recommendations to attending physicians decreased unnecessary polypharmacy, incorrect dosing, and potential drug-drug and drug-disease interactions by 36% relative to usual care.[56] The remainder of this section highlights a few approaches that can help efforts to optimize medication management in older adults.

Medication Review

A critical first step in addressing polypharmacy is to obtain an accurate list of current medications that includes both prescription and over-the-counter medications. This can often be challenging, especially when a patient has multiple providers, uses multiple pharmacies, has recently had transitions in care site (eg, hospitalized), and has comorbid conditions that impact cognitive and physical function. Despite clinicians' best efforts, there are often discrepancies between what patients are actually taking and what is recorded in the medical record. A "brown bag" review, in which patients bring in all of their medicines (prescription and nonprescription) to their appointment, is a critical "procedure" for primary care providers to carry out. Calls to pharmacies and review of medications by home health nurses and family are often necessary to confirm ongoing medication use. Clinic visits should intermittently include "brown bag" reviews with much or all of an appointment devoted to considering each medication and whether it is effective, tolerated, and still appropriate for the patient to be taking. One study of potentially remediable adverse drug events found that 63% were attributable to the physician's failure to respond to medication-related symptoms and 37% were related to the patient's failure to inform the physician of the symptoms.[57] Such data suggest that "brown bag" reviews could help reduce adverse drug events by helping to foster increased communication about each medicine the patient is taking.

Avoid the Prescribing Cascade

The prescribing cascade refers to when an adverse effect of one drug is misinterpreted as a new medical condition that leads to prescription of another drug.[58] The result is added unnecessary medications that add to patient's medication burden and increase the risk of polypharmacy. Examples of prescribing cascades include the following:

- Hydrochlorothiazide → ↑ uric acid → gout → allopurinol rx
- NSAIDs → ↑ salt retention/renal effects → ↑ blood pressure → antihypertensives
- Metoclopramide → extrapyramidal side effects → carbidopa/levodopa
- Cholinesterase inhibitors → ↑ cholinergic activity at bladder → oxybutynin (of note, this combination also may decrease the already modest efficacy of the cholinesterase inhibitor)

Before initiating a new prescription, clinicians should always ask the question "is this new medication possibly being used to treat effects of another drug?"

Opportunities to Stop Medications

Although providers always should be vigilant about revisiting the risks and benefits of medications in older adults, there are certain times when such reviews are especially appropriate (**Box 4**). Transitions in care represent an important time to revisit medications, as usually the need to go to/from home to a hospital, rehabilitation, or other care setting implies that health status has changed. Such changes may extend to physical and cognitive function as well as patient preferences. Further, medication errors are frequent during transitions in care, providing further reason for scrutiny of medications

---
Box 4
Opportunities to revisit/stop medications

- Whenever writing a new prescription (eg, can an existing medication be stopped to keep drug burden neutral?)
- At a scheduled annual/semiannual medication review "brown bag" appointment
- Care transitions are key opportunities
  - Is the patient managing current care plan?
  - Is drug complexity impacting adherence and safety?
  - Have patient preferences changed?

---

at these times.[59] One study found that nearly one-half of hospitalized patients were prescribed at least 1 unnecessary drug at the time of discharge from the hospital, providing further rationale for extra attention to medication review and reconciliation.[60] Common culprits include PPIs, benzodiazepines, and vitamin and mineral supplements.[6,61,62]

Providers may be reluctant to discontinue medications owing to concerns regarding worsening of underlying disease or rebound/withdrawal effects. Such concerns are appropriate, as in one study of 124 ambulatory older outpatients, 26% of drug discontinuations were accompanied by worsening of the underlying disease (eg, recurrent angina or elevated blood pressure) and roughly 10% of discontinuations resulted in hospitalization, or emergency department or urgent care clinic visits.[63] Accordingly, providers should be vigilant about disease recurrence and educate patients about the need to report relevant signs and symptoms after medication discontinuation. Still, most (74%) medication discontinuations were well tolerated and it is possible that drug reductions resulted in decreased health care use among the persons who reduced their medication burden. For example, one study conducted in elderly nursing home residents found that a drug reduction intervention that led to stopping, on average, 3 of 7 medications led to decreased hospitalization and mortality rates.[64] The same intervention among older outpatients stopped, on average, 4 of 8 medications, and only 2% of drugs were restarted due to recurrence of the original indication. Further, no significant adverse events or deaths were attributable to discontinuation, and 88% of patients reported global improvement in health.[65]

General rules to consider when stopping medications include the following:

- Slowly taper medications to discontinuation, especially medications that interact with receptors, for which abrupt discontinuation may result in rebound or symptom flare (eg, β-blockers, SSRIs, opioids, benzodiazepines).[6]
- Communicate medication changes made in the hospital or other care settings to the primary care provider to avoid medication errors as patients move through care transitions.
- Communicate medication discontinuations to the patient's pharmacy. One study found that it is not uncommon for patients to still refill and take medications that have been discontinued. This problem may relate to electronic prescribing that may not include directives to the pharmacy to discontinue refills of medications that have been electronically stopped or altered.[66]

Match Drug Regimens to Patient Conditions and Goals of Care

The optimal approach to medication prescribing is patient-centered and takes into account the patient's current condition and longer-term goals of care. This is especially important in older adults with multiple medical conditions, where a disease-focused approach often leads to polypharmacy, unclear benefits, and possibly harm. Patients' feelings and beliefs about their health, medical conditions, and treatment options also are key factors in whether or not they will adhere to prescribed medications.[19] Factors such as prognosis, time to benefit, and potential adverse effects become increasingly important with advancing age. Further, these factors and patient preferences may change over time. Clinicians should engage patients in discussions about goals, especially when following guidelines. For example, a typical question to discuss with a patient with coronary artery disease might be the following: Will the addition of a β-blocker and statin as part of an 11-drug regimen provide greater benefit than harm to an older patient whose priorities may be maximal energy, strength, and sense of well-being in favor of a reduced risk of heart attack or stroke over the next 5 years?[8] Questions that patients and clinicians should consider when prescribing medications for older adults include the following:

- Is the drug being considered clearly indicated and effective based on studies that included persons similar to this patient?
- What are the therapeutic end points?
- Do the benefits outweigh the risks?
- Is it used to treat side effects of another drug?
- Could it interact with underlying diseases or other drugs in the regimen?
- Consider compliance and cost challenges
- Does the patient know the indication for the drug, how to take it, and what adverse effects to look for?

1. Accurately ascertain all current drug use
- 'brown paper bag' medication reconciliation

2. Identify patients at risk of, or suffering, ADR
- at risk: ≥8 medications
  advanced age (>75 years)
  high-risk medications
- assess for current, past or highly likely future toxicity

  All three at-risk criteria – aim for ≤ 5 drugs
  Discontinue drugs for which there is unequivoval
  evidence of past, current or future toxicity
  (eg triple whammy of NSAID, diuretic, ACE inhibitor)

3. Estimate life expectancy
- clinical prognostication tools or lifespan calculators

4. Define overall care goals
- consider current functional status and quality of life with
  reference to estimated life expectancy

  If life expectancy less than 2 years, preservation of
  function and quality of life predominate over
  prolonging life and avoiding future complications as
  goals of care

5. Verify current indications for ongoing treatments
- perform diagnosis-medication reconciliation
- confirm diagnostic labels against formal diagnostic criteria
- ascertain, for each confirmed diagnosis, drug appropriateness

  Discontinue drugs for which the diagnosis is wrong or
  totally unsubstantiated or where, for a confirmed
  diagnosis, the drug is ineffective

6. Determine need for disease-specific preventive medications
- estimate clinical impact and time to future treatment benefit
- compare this estimate with expected lifespan

  Discontinue preventive drugs whose time until benefit
  exceeds expected lifespan

7. Determine absolute benefit-harm thresholds of medications
- reconcile estimates of absolute benefit and harm using prediction
  tools (see http://www.mdcalc.com)

  Discontinue drugs whose absolute level of harm
  exceeds absolute level of benefit; in 'line-ball' cases
  elicit patient preferences

8. Review the relative utility of individual drugs
- rank drugs according to the relative utility from high to low based on
  predicted benefit, harm, administration and monitoring burden

  Discontinue drugs of low utility

9. Identify drugs to be discontinued and seek patient consent
- reconcile drugs for discontinuation with patient preferences

  Discontinue drugs patients are not in favor of taking

10. Devise and implement drug discontinuation plan with close monitoring

Fig. 2. Algorithm to optimize medication use in older adults. (*From* Scott AI, Gray LC, Martin JH, et al. Deciding when to stop: toward evidence-based deprescribing of drugs in older populations. Evid Based Med 2013;18(4):122; with permission.)

Fig. 2 provides an algorithmic approach to improving medication use modeled after a 10-step conceptual framework proposed by Scott and colleagues.[67]

SUMMARY

Older adults often receive inappropriate medications and experience the vast majority of adverse drug events. The problem is especially challenging in older adults with multiple medical conditions and frailty, for whom risks from medications may be greater and benefits less certain. Tools and expert recommendations are available in the literature to help guide providers in their efforts to optimize drug therapy in older adults. As long-term management of multiple chronic diseases among an increasingly older population becomes the face of modern medicine, the rational use of medications (and other available interventions) remains a challenge to be appropriately addressed.

REFERENCES

1. Qato DM, Alexander GC, Conti RM, et al. Use of prescription and over-the-counter medications and dietary supplements among older adults in the United States. JAMA 2008;300(24):2867–78.
2. Brahma DK, Wahlang JB, Marak MD, et al. Adverse drug reactions in the elderly. J Pharmacol Pharmacother 2013;4(2):91–4.
3. Gnjidic D, Hilmer SN, Blyth FM, et al. Polypharmacy cutoff and outcomes: five or more medicines were used to identify community-dwelling older men at risk of different adverse outcomes. J Clin Epidemiol 2012;65(9):989–95.
4. Onder G, Petrovic M, Tangiisuran B, et al. Development and validation of a score to assess risk of adverse drug reactions among in-hospital patients 65 years or older: the GerontoNet ADR risk score. Arch Intern Med 2010;170(13):1142.
5. Kaufman DW, Kelly JP, Rosenberg L, et al. Recent patterns of medication use in the ambulatory adult population of the United States: the Slone survey. JAMA 2002;287:337–44.
6. Steinman MA, Hanlon JT. Managing medications in clinically complex elders: "There's got to be a happy medium." JAMA 2010;304(14):1592–601.
7. Boyd CM, Darer J, Boult C, et al. Clinical practice guidelines and quality of care for older patients with multiple comorbid diseases: implications for pay for performance. JAMA 2005;294:716.
8. Tinetti ME, Bogardus ST Jr, Agostini JV. Potential pitfalls of disease-specific guidelines for patients with multiple conditions. N Engl J Med 2004;351(27):2870–4.
9. Zarowitz B, Stebelsky L, Muma B, et al. Reduction of high-risk polypharmacy drug combinations in patients in a managed care setting. Pharmacotherapy 2005;25(11):1636–45.
10. American Geriatrics Society Expert Panel on the Care of Older Adults with Multimorbidity. Patient-centered care for older adults with multiple chronic conditions: a stepwise approach from the American Geriatrics Society: American Geriatrics Society Expert Panel on the Care of Older Adults with Multimorbidity. J Am Geriatr Soc 2012;60(10):1957–68.
11. Mannucci PM, Nobili A, REPOSI Investigators. Multimorbidity and polypharmacy in the elderly: lessons from REPOSI. Intern Emerg Med 2014;9:723–34.
12. The American Geriatrics Society 2012 Beers Criteria Update Expert Panel. American Geriatrics Society updated Beers Criteria for potentially inappropriate medication use in older adults. J Am Geriatr Soc 2012;60:616–31.
13. HEDIS. Available at: http://www.ncqa.org/tabid/1274/default.aspx. Accessed October 3, 2014.

14. Budnitz DS, Lovegrove MC, Shehab N, et al. Emergency hospitalizations for adverse drug events in older Americans. N Engl J Med 2011;365:2002–12.
15. You JJ, Singer DE, Howard PA, et al. Antithrombotic therapy for atrial fibrillation: antithrombotic therapy and prevention of thrombosis, 9th ed: American College of Chest Physicians evidence-based clinical practice guidelines. Chest 2012;141: 531S.
16. Hurlen M, Abdelnoor M, Smith P, et al. Warfarin, aspirin, or both after myocardial infarction. N Engl J Med 2002;347(13):969–74.
17. WHO. Adherence to long-term therapies. World Health Organization; 2003. Available at: http://www.who.int/chp/knowledge/publications/adherence_report/en/. Accessed October 3, 2014.
18. Chang TI, Desai M, Solomon DH, et al. Kidney function and long-term medication adherence after myocardial infarction in the elderly. Clin J Am Soc Nephrol 2011; 6(4):864–9.
19. Osterberg L, Blaschke T. Adherence to medication. N Engl J Med 2005;353(5): 487–97.
20. Coleman CI, Limone B, Sobieraj DM, et al. Dosing frequency and medication adherence in chronic disease. J Manag Care Pharm 2012;18:527.
21. Choudhry NK, Fischer MA, Avorn J, et al. The implications of therapeutic complexity on adherence to cardiovascular medications. Arch Intern Med 2011;171:814–22.
22. Glasheen JJ, Fugit RV, Prochazka AV. The risk of overanticoagulation with antibiotic use in outpatients on stable warfarin regimens. J Gen Intern Med 2005;20(7): 653–6.
23. Hylek EM, Heiman H, Skates SJ, et al. Acetaminophen and other risk factors for excessive warfarin anticoagulation. JAMA 1998;279(9):657–62.
24. Mahe I, Bertrand N, Droeut L, et al. Interaction between paracetamol and warfarin in patients: a double-blind, placebo-controlled, randomized study. Haematologica 2006;91(12):1621–7.
25. Zhang Q, Bal-dit-Sollier C, Droeut L, et al. Interaction between acetaminophen and warfarin in adults receiving long-term oral anticoagulants: a randomized controlled trial. Eur J Clin Pharmacol 2011;67:309–14.
26. Centanni M, Gargano L, Canettieri G, et al. Thyroxine in goiter, *Helicobacter pylori* infection, and chronic gastritis. N Engl J Med 2006;354:1787–95.
27. Derendorf H, VanderMaelen CP, Brickl RS, et al. Dipyridamole bioavailability in subjects with reduced gastric acidity. J Clin Pharmacol 2005;45:845–50.
28. Lehner E, Annibale B, Delle Fave G. Systematic review: impaired drug absorption related to the co-administration of antisecretory therapy. Aliment Pharmacol Ther 2009;29:1219–29.
29. Mahabaleshwarkar RK, Yang Y, Datar MV, et al. Risk of adverse cardiovascular outcomes and all-cause mortality associated with concomitant use of clopidogrel and proton pump inhibitors in elderly patients. Curr Med Res Opin 2013;29(4):315–23.
30. Chen J, Chen SY, Lian JJ. Pharmacodynamic impacts of proton pump inhibitors on the efficacy of clopidogrel in vivo–a systematic review. Clin Cardiol 2013;36(4): 184–9.
31. Depta JP, Lenzini PA, Lanfear DE. Clinical outcomes associated with proton pump inhibitor use among clopidogrel-treated patients within CYP2C19 genotype groups following acute myocardial infarction. Pharmacogenomics J 2014. [Epub ahead of print].
32. Johnson DA, Chilton R, Liker HR. Proton-pump inhibitors in patients requiring antiplatelet therapy: new FDA labeling. Postgrad Med 2014;126(3):239–45.

33. O'Connell MB, Madden DM, Murray AM. Effects of proton pump inhibitors on calcium carbonate absorption in women: a randomized crossover trial. Am J Med 2005;118(7):778–81.
34. Ngamruengphong S, Leontiadis GI, Radhi S, et al. Proton pump inhibitors and risk of fracture: a systematic review and meta-analysis of observational studies. Am J Gastroenterol 2011;106:1209–18.
35. Yu EW, Bauer SR, Bain PA, et al. Proton pump inhibitors and risk of fractures: a meta-analysis of 11 international studies. Am J Med 2011;124:519–26.
36. Corleto VD, Festaa S, Di Giulioa E, et al. Proton pump inhibitor therapy and potential long-term harm. Curr Opin Endocrinol Diabetes Obes 2014;21:3–8.
37. Stabler S. Clinical practice: vitamin B12 deficiency. N Engl J Med 2013;368(2):149–60.
38. Kellick KA, Bottorff M, Toth PP. A clinician's guide to statin drug-drug interactions. J Clin Lipidol 2014;8:S30–46.
39. Gandhi S, Fleet JL, Bailey DG, et al. Calcium-channel blocker–clarithromycin drug interactions and acute kidney injury. JAMA 2013;310(23):2544–53.
40. Wright AJ, Gomes T, Mamdani MM, et al. The risk of hypotension following co-prescription of macrolide antibiotics and calcium-channel blockers. CMAJ 2011;183(3):303–7.
41. Jacob S, Spinler SA. Hyponatremia associated with selective serotonin-reuptake inhibitors in older adults. Ann Pharmacother 2006;40(9):1618–22.
42. Krüger S, Lindstaedt M. Duloxetine and hyponatremia: a report of 5 cases. J Clin Psychopharmacol 2007;27(1):101–4.
43. Grover S, Somaiya M, Ghormode D. Venlafaxine-associated hyponatremia presenting with catatonia. J Neuropsychiatry Clin Neurosci 2013;25(2):E11–2.
44. Dirks AC, van Hyfte DM. Recurrent hyponatremia after substitution of citalopram with duloxetine. J Clin Psychopharmacol 2007;27(3):313.
45. Jiang HY, Chen HZ, Hu XJ, et al. Use of selective serotonin reuptake inhibitors and risk of upper gastrointestinal bleeding: a systematic review and meta-analysis. Clin Gastroenterol Hepatol 2015;13(1):42–50.
46. Anglin R, Yuan Y, Moayyedi P, et al. Risk of upper gastrointestinal bleeding with selective serotonin reuptake inhibitors with or without concurrent nonsteroidal anti-inflammatory use: a systematic review and meta-analysis. Am J Gastroenterol 2014;109(6):811–9.
47. Wang YP, Chen YT, Tsai CF, et al. Short-term use of serotonin reuptake inhibitors and risk of upper gastrointestinal bleeding. Am J Psychiatry 2014;171(1):54–61.
48. van Walraven C, Mamdani MM, Wells PS. Inhibition of serotonin reuptake by antidepressants and upper gastrointestinal bleeding in elderly patients: retrospective cohort study. BMJ 2001;323(7314):655–8.
49. Stahlmann R, Lode H. Safety considerations of fluoroquinolones in the elderly: an update. Drugs Aging 2010;27(3):193–209.
50. Wise BL, Peloquin C, Choi H. Impact of age, sex, obesity, and steroid use on quinolone-associated tendon disorders. Am J Med 2012;125(12):1228–34.
51. Fluoroquinolones and peripheral neuropathy. Med Lett Drugs Ther 2013;55(1429):89.
52. Antoniou T, Gomes T, Juurlink DN, et al. Trimethoprim-sulfamethoxazole–induced hyperkalemia in patients receiving inhibitors of the renin-angiotensin system. Arch Intern Med 2010;170(12):1045–9.
53. Witt JM, Koo JM, Danielson BD. Effect of standard-dose trimethoprim/sulfamethoxazole on the serum potassium concentration in elderly men. Ann Pharmacother 1996;30(4):347–50.

54. Gnjidic D, Le Couteur DG, Kouladjian L, et al. Deprescribing trials: methods to reduce polypharmacy and the impact on prescribing and clinical outcomes. Clin Geriatr Med 2012;28(2):237–53.

55. Barry PJ, Gallagher P, Ryan C, et al. (Screening tool to alert doctors to the right treatment)–an evidence-based screening tool to detect prescribing omissions in elderly patients. Age Ageing 2007;36:632–8.

56. Gallagher PF, O'Connor MN, O'Mahony D. Prevention of potentially inappropriate prescribing for elderly patients: a randomized controlled trial using STOPP/START criteria. Clin Pharmacol Ther 2011;89(6):845–54.

57. Gandhi TK, Weingart SN, Borus J, et al. Adverse drug events in ambulatory care. N Engl J Med 2003;348(16):1556–64.

58. Rochon PA, Gurwitz JH. Optimising drug treatment for elderly people: the prescribing cascade. BMJ 1997;315:1096–9.

59. Sinvani LD, Beizer J, Akerman M, et al. Medication reconciliation in continuum of care transitions: a moving target. J Am Med Dir Assoc 2013;14:668–72.

60. Hajjar ER, Hanlon JT, Sloane RJ, et al. Unnecessary drug use in frail older people at hospital discharge. J Am Geriatr Soc 2005;53(9):1518–23.

61. Halme AS, Beland SG, Preville M, et al. Uncovering the source of new benzodiazepine prescriptions in community-dwelling older adults. Int J Geriatr Psychiatry 2013;28(3):248–55.

62. Grant K, Al-Adhami N, Tordoff J, et al. Continuation of proton pump inhibitors from hospital to community. Pharm World Sci 2006;28(4):189–93.

63. Graves T, Hanlon JT, Schmader KE, et al. Adverse events after discontinuing medications in elderly outpatients. Arch Intern Med 1997;157(19):2205–10.

64. Garfinkel D, Zur-Gil S, Ben-Israel J. The war against polypharmacy: a new cost-effective geriatric-palliative approach for improving drug therapy in disabled elderly people. Isr Med Assoc J 2007;9(6):430–4.

65. Garfinkel D, Mangin D. Feasibility study of a systematic approach for discontinuation of multiple medications in older adults: addressing polypharmacy. Arch Intern Med 2010;170(18):1648–54.

66. Allen AS, Sequist TD. Pharmacy dispensing of electronically discontinued medications. Ann Intern Med 2012;157:700–5.

67. Scott AI, Gray LC, Martin JH, et al. Deciding when to stop: towards evidence-based deprescribing of drugs in older populations. Evid Based Med 2013;18(4):121–4.

Evaluation and Management of the Elderly Patient Presenting with Cognitive Complaints

Kerry L. Hildreth, MD*, Skotti Church, MD

KEYWORDS

• Cognitive impairment • Dementia • Alzheimer disease • Elderly

KEY POINTS

• Cognitive complaints in elderly patients are common and may range from normal aging to dementia; complaints should always be evaluated rather than be attributed to aging.

• Cognitive impairment in elderly patients is often multifactorial, and potential roles of medications, depression, delirium, alcohol use, and other comorbid conditions should be considered.

• Dementia is a clinical diagnosis, with laboratory and imaging studies used to eliminate other explanations for the impairments.

• Management goals for patients with cognitive complaints center on preserving function and quality of life, advance care planning, and caregiver support; goals will change with progression of disease.

• Although no pharmacologic or nonpharmacologic therapies have been shown to alter the progression of Alzheimer dementia, they may modestly improve symptoms in some patients.

INTRODUCTION

Cognitive complaints in elderly patients may arise from the patient or from family, friends, or caregivers. Any cognitive complaint, regardless of the source, should be investigated rather than attributed to aging. Although current recommendations do not recommend for or against routine screening for cognitive impairment in geriatric patients,[1] many geriatric practitioners routinely assess cognitive function, especially as the Medicare Annual Wellness Visit now requires a cognitive assessment.[2]

The authors have no disclosures to report.
Division of Geriatric Medicine, University of Colorado School of Medicine, 12631 East 17th Avenue, Room 8111, Aurora, CO 80045, USA
* Corresponding author.
E-mail address: kerry.hildreth@ucdenver.edu

Med Clin N Am 99 (2015) 311–335
http://dx.doi.org/10.1016/j.mcna.2014.11.006
0025-7125/15/$ – see front matter © 2015 Elsevier Inc. All rights reserved.

Despite increased awareness and education about the most common type of dementia, Alzheimer disease (AD), many patients and families are unsure which cognitive changes are normal and which may signal a more serious problem. Age-associated memory impairment (AAMI) is a term used to broadly define normal age-related cognitive changes, including difficulty recalling specific details or dates of past events (episodic memory), difficulty multitasking, and slower processing speed for new learning or "working" memory. AAMI may occur as early as age 50 years and is not associated with progression to dementia or an underlying disease state. Most importantly, changes resulting from AAMI should not affect functional abilities.

Subjective cognitive impairment is a relatively new construct whereby patients perceive deficits that are not detectable with objective measures. However, some data suggest that patients with subjective cognitive impairment are at increased risk of developing objective deficits over time.[3,4] Mild cognitive impairment (MCI) is defined as objective cognitive impairment with preserved function.[5] MCI has historically been a controversial entity with significant clinical heterogeneity. Estimates of the conversion rate to dementia (usually AD) in patients with MCI vary, but appear to be approximately 10% per year, compared with 1% to 3% per year in cognitively normal older adults.[6–8] However, many patients with MCI remain stable over time, and some studies have shown improvement in a substantial proportion of patients.[8–10] Whether MCI is in fact prodromal AD has thus been debated. Recent efforts have focused on distinguishing MCI due to AD from that attributable to other causes to facilitate clinical utility.[11] The feature that separates dementia from MCI is the effect of the impairment on daily function. In dementia the impairments affect daily function, whereas in MCI they do not.[12]

EVALUATION
Patient History

As with many geriatric conditions, cognitive impairment is frequently multifactorial; thus, a detailed history is critical (**Table 1**). Even though truly reversible causes of dementia are exceedingly rare, multiple factors such as medications, depression, delirium, infections, alcohol use, or metabolic disorders may exacerbate underlying cognitive impairment. Addressing possible contributing factors may significantly improve cognitive symptoms even though the underlying disease process cannot be treated.

In addition to the timing and progression of symptoms, specific examples of deficits should be elicited from the patient and a reliable informant. Ideally the patient and informant are interviewed separately, as informants may hesitate to contradict the patient or describe episodes or symptoms that may be embarrassing to the patient. Directed questions about changes in handling finances, participation in hobbies or activities, and driving abilities can help assess the severity of complaints. Specific inquiries about safety are essential, as these require immediate action. As older adults with cognitive impairment are at high risk for physical abuse, neglect, and financial exploitation, knowledge of the patient's living situation, care providers, and the caregiver's capabilities and support network is imperative.

Traditional cardiometabolic risk factors such as diabetes, hypertension, obesity, and dyslipidemia are strongly linked to the development of cognitive impairment and dementia, including AD.[13] A history of cerebrovascular disease or neurologic disorder (eg, multiple sclerosis, amyotrophic lateral sclerosis, Parkinson disease) may suggest an underlying cause in other cases. As with any geriatric syndrome, a complete review of all medications, including over-the-counter products, vitamins, supplements, and herbal remedies, should be part of the evaluation.

Table 1
Key elements of cognitive impairment history

History of present illness	Details, timing, and progression of complaints
	Corroboration from a reliable informant
	Functional status (basic and instrumental ADLs)
	Safety (driving, appliances, firearms, wandering, finances)
Medical history	Cardiovascular diseases or risk factors
	Chronic neurologic diseases
	History of head trauma or concussions
	Recent illness or hospitalizations
Social history	Current living situation and support network
	Past or present substance use/abuse
	Recent relocation, life events, losses
Medication review	Benzodiazepines
	Anticholinergic/antimuscarinic agents
	Sedative hypnotics
	Tricyclic antidepressants
	Opioids
	Anticonvulsants
Review of systems	Mood or behavioral disturbances, personality changes
	Focal neurologic symptoms (sensory or motor complaints, headaches, seizure activity, tremor, gait impairment)
	Incontinence
	Sleep disturbance

Abbreviation: ADLs, activities of daily livings.

Delirium should be considered, especially in patients who have recently been hospitalized. Delirium is distinguished from other causes of cognitive impairment by the acute time course, association with a specific stressor such as an infection or medication effect, and marked inattention. However, it is well recognized that delirium may persist for weeks to months, and that an episode of delirium may unmask previously unrecognized dementia.[14]

Patients with cognitive complaints should be asked about a history of depression and about current depressive symptoms. The relation between depression and dementia is complex; a history of depression increases the risk of developing dementia, and depression itself can cause significant cognitive impairment that may mimic dementia. Furthermore, depression is a common feature of dementia, present in approximately 50% of patients with AD,[15] especially in early-stage disease when significant insight into the disease process may exist.

Pathophysiology

The wide clinical spectrum of cognitive impairment and dementia reflects the interplay of neuropathology, cerebral metabolism, synaptic failure, and inflammation that result in temporary or permanent cognitive decline. Regardless of the specific underlying pathology, which is often poorly understood, the final common pathway in dementia is neuronal death and cell loss, as evidenced by correlations between atrophy and dementia across all ages.[16] The clinical presentation reflects the affected regions of the brain. Cognitive complaints tend to stem from damage to the cerebral cortex; subcortical injury can also cause cognitive impairment, but is often associated with psychiatric or motor symptoms.

The pathophysiology of AD has been the most intensively studied to date. There are likely multiple mechanisms and pathways leading to the initiation and progression of AD, but most research to date has centered on the neuropathologic hallmarks required for definitive diagnosis, amyloid plaques, and neurofibrillary tangles. Though controversial, the amyloid hypothesis of AD has dominated AD research since it was proposed in the early 1990s.[17] According to the amyloid hypothesis, it is the accumulation and aggregation of misfolded β-amyloid peptide (Aβ) that initiates and perpetuates neurodegeneration in AD. Cleavage of the amyloid precursor protein produces Aβ, which aggregates into toxic oligomers.[18] Over time these oligomers merge into insoluble fibrils and, eventually, the characteristic plaques of AD.

Neurofibrillary tangles consist of aggregations of abnormally hyperphosphorylated tau proteins, which self-aggregate to form paired helical filaments and, eventually, tangles.[18] This process destabilizes microtubules, impairing axonal transport and resulting in neuronal dysfunction and degeneration.[18] Tau accumulation, or tauopathy, is also a feature of frontotemporal and subcortical dementias.[19]

Vascular contributions to AD are an active area of research. Approximately 60% to 90% of patients with AD have ischemic disease, and up to one-third of presumed cases of vascular dementia exhibit the neuropathologic features of AD.[18] Some have suggested that better management of modifiable cardiovascular risk factors may be partly responsible for the recently observed decrease in the prevalence and incidence of age-specific dementia.[20]

Physical Examination

The physical examination may be completely normal in many patients with cognitive complaints. The patient's general appearance may offer some clues as to possibility of the cause and severity of the cognitive complaint. For example, delirious patients may show signs of either psychomotor agitation or slowing. Patients with either dementia or depression may show signs of self-neglect or poor hygiene. A thorough neurologic examination should be performed to detect any focal deficits, Parkinsonian signs, upper motor neuron signs, or gait disturbance that may indicate a potential underlying process and guide further evaluation and testing. Frontal release signs (eg, grasp, palmomental, snout, glabellar reflexes) are typically present only in advanced dementia.

Cognitive Testing

Administration of a structured cognitive assessment tool is recommended in any elderly patient with a cognitive complaint. Many tools are suitable for use in a primary care setting, and no single test is clearly superior. Considerations in selecting a test include time, education level, language barriers, severity of deficits, and cognitive domains of interest (**Table 2**). Performance on cognitive assessments may sometimes provide clues to the underlying etiology. For example, patients with depression may exhibit inattention and poor motivation. Patients with AD may have marked loss of short-term memory and executive function, whereas impairments primarily in language may point toward frontotemporal dementia.

Neuropsychiatric Symptoms

Neuropsychiatric symptoms such as depression, anxiety, irritability, and agitation are common, developing in 90% of patients with dementia within 5 years of diagnosis (**Fig. 1**).[15] Frequently these symptoms precede the diagnosis of dementia, and can be helpful in pointing toward a cause in some cases. Prominent neuropsychiatric findings or behavioral problems on initial evaluation may suggest cognitive impairment

Table 2
Common brief cognitive screening tools

Test	Time (min)	Advantages	Limitations
Mini-Mental Status Examination[118] (MMSE)	7–10	Most widely used and studied worldwide Often used as a reference for comparative evaluations of other assessments Required for some drug insurance reimbursements	Education/age/language/ culture bias Ceiling effect (highly educated impaired subjects pass) Proprietary: unless used from memory, test needs to be purchased Best performance for at least moderate cognitive impairment
Montreal Cognitive Assessment[119] (MoCA)	10–15	Designed to test for mild cognitive impairment Multiple languages accessible Tests many separate domains (7)	Lacks studies in general practice settings Education bias (≤ 12 y) Limited use and evidence: published data are relatively new (2005) Administration time ≥ 10 min
St Louis University Mental Status Examination[120] (SLUMS)	7	No education bias Tests many separate domains (7)	Limited use and evidence: published data are relatively new (2006) Studied in Veterans Affairs geriatric clinic (predominantly white males)
Mini-Cog[121]	2–4	Developed for and validated in primary care and multiple languages/cultures Little or no education/ language/race bias Short administration time	Use of different word lists may affect failure rates Some study results based on longer tests with the Mini-Cog elements reviewed independently

Adapted from Cordell CB, Borson S, Boustani M, et al. Alzheimer's Association recommendations for operationalizing the detection of cognitive impairment during the Medicare Annual Wellness Visit in a primary care setting. Alzheimers Dement 2013;9(2):147. http://dx.doi.org/10.1016/ j.jalz.2012.09.011; with permission.

resulting from non-AD dementias. Disinhibition and personality changes with relatively preserved memory and executive function are characteristic of frontotemporal dementias. Visual hallucinations and delusions paired with motor abnormalities are often seen in Lewy body dementia (LBD).

Imaging and Additional Testing

At present there are no laboratory tests or imaging studies that definitively diagnose dementia in the clinical setting. Although significant progress has been made in identifying biomarkers for AD, particularly amyloid imaging and cerebrospinal fluid (CSF) markers, these tests are not sufficiently standardized or widely available outside of research settings. Basic laboratory testing is recommended to evaluate for metabolic and other disorders that may cause or contribute to cognitive impairment, including complete blood count, comprehensive metabolic panel, thyroid function testing, and vitamin B_{12}. Testing for human immunodeficiency virus and neurosyphilis can

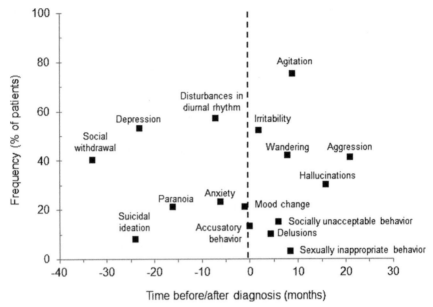

Fig. 1. Frequency and timing of behavioral disturbances in Alzheimer disease. (*From* Ballard CG, Gauthier S, Cummings JL, et al. Management of agitation and aggression associated with Alzheimer disease. Nat Rev Neurol 2009;5(5):246; with permission.)

be considered in individuals at risk, but are not recommended as part of the routine evaluation.

The American Academy of Neurology recommends obtaining a noncontrast head computed tomography (CT) or MRI scan as part of the initial evaluation of cognitive impairment[21]; however, in primary care practice this decision is often guided instead by the presenting signs and symptoms, and the likelihood that imaging will provide useful information. For example, in patients with focal neurologic deficits, recent head trauma, or neurologic complaints such as headache, imaging may help identify or eliminate other possible causes of the cognitive complaints. Patients in whom the cognitive complaints are acute, rapidly progressive, or atypical should also receive imaging with the choice of modality depending on availability and suspicion for causes such as hemorrhage or mass lesions for which CT would be sufficient. Conversely, in patients with moderate to severe dementia and a typical clinical presentation and progression, imaging is unlikely to be useful. In patients with dementia, neuroimaging may be normal, or show global or focal atrophy. Findings of cortical or subcortical infarcts or a high burden of chronic small-vessel disease may suggest a vascular cause, and the location may correlate with the clinical presentation. Functional MRI and PET imaging are additional imaging modalities being studied for use in the diagnosis of dementia. These techniques may better elucidate the pathophysiology of cognitive impairment and dementia, but, as with amyloid imaging, they are not currently recommended for the evaluation of cognitive complaints.[21]

Lumbar puncture and CSF analysis is not recommended in the standard workup of cognitive impairment, but may be helpful in rapidly progressive or atypical dementias. Genetic testing is likewise not routinely performed. To date, the only gene identified as increasing susceptibility to late-onset, sporadic AD, which accounts for greater than

95% of cases, is the apolipoprotein (*APOE*)-*ε4* allele. Although heterozygosity and homozygosity for *APOE-ε4* increase the risk of AD by approximately 2-fold and 10-fold, respectively, it is neither necessary nor sufficient for the development of AD. In rare cases of strongly familial early-onset disease, referral for genetic testing for identified mutations in the processing of amyloid precursor protein may be considered.[22]

Diagnostic Dilemmas

A general algorithm for the evaluation of cognitive complaints in older adults is presented in **Fig. 2**. Uncertainty about the diagnosis, or atypical presentations such as early onset (<65 years), rapid progression ($\leq$6 months), or isolated cognitive deficits should prompt referral for neurologic and/or psychological evaluation. Less common types of dementia (eg, prion disease, autoimmune, infectious, neoplastic) may require specialized diagnostic and management skills. Formal neuropsychological testing can be informative in cases where psychiatric disease is suggested, or for suspected impairment in highly educated individuals who may score within the normal range on standard assessments despite significant deficits. These sensitive and detailed assessments can also provide anticipatory guidance and compensatory strategies for patients and families, and facilitate reevaluation, tracking of disease progression, and prognostic guidance in some cases.

PATIENT MANAGEMENT
Management Goals

For all patients with cognitive complaints, primary goals include maintaining function and independence, preventing further cognitive decline, and ensuring quality of life. Depending on the presumed cause and the severity of impairment, specific goals and strategies will vary significantly. The management of cognitive impairment is unique in that the caregiver is a critical part of the alliance between patient and provider, and must be highly involved and supported for successful attainment of goals.

Subjective cognitive impairment
For patients with only subjective cognitive complaints, the goals are reassurance, optimizing management of any comorbid conditions, and promoting a healthy lifestyle. However, these patients should be monitored carefully for any signs of progression, as studies have suggested that subjective cognitive impairment is predictive of future MCI.[3,4]

Mild cognitive impairment
An important goal for patients with MCI is acceptance of the uncertainty surrounding this diagnosis given the possibility of progression, stability, or even improvement. Collaboration with the health care provider and utilization of community resources such as the Alzheimer's Association for support and education can help patients and caregivers manage the inevitable frustration and fear associated with this diagnosis.

Careful attention to the management of comorbid conditions that may worsen cognitive impairment (eg, depression, heart failure, sleep apnea, hypertension, diabetes) should be part of the management plan, particularly with respect to the management of vascular risk factors. Clinicians should conduct a rigorous and ongoing review of all prescription and nonprescription medications that may affect cognition, and consider alternatives when possible. Impairments in memory and executive function may affect adherence to medications and treatment plans; regimens should be simplified and other methods, such as automated medication dispensers, pill boxes,

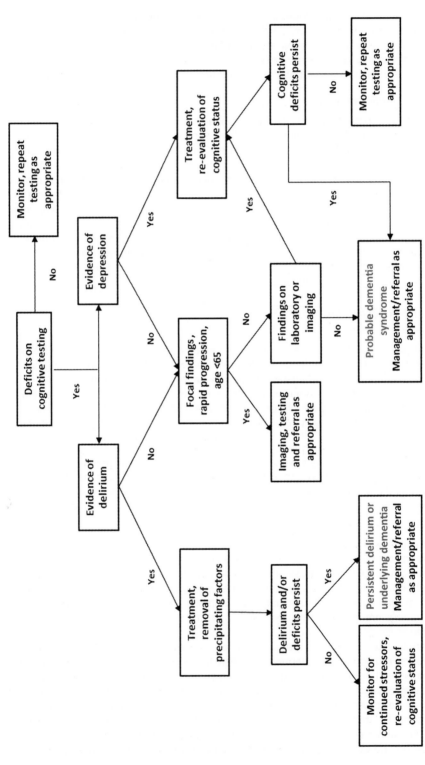

Fig. 2. Algorithm for the evaluation of cognitive complaints in elderly adults.

and caregiver oversight should be considered to help prevent errors. Patients should be encouraged to remain physically, socially, and intellectually active while realizing that their usual activities may need to be modified to compensate for cognitive deficits. The caregiver's physical and mental health need to be monitored and supported, so assessment of the caregiver's level of ability and understanding of the disease are essential.

Although many patients with MCI remain stable over time, the risk of progression to dementia, usually AD, is significantly higher than in cognitively normal older adults.[6–8] Thus, establishing a safety net and advance care planning are important. Ideally, patients and caregivers will discuss potential issues such as driving, eventual need for a higher level of care (eg, home care, assisted living), financial planning, and end-of-life goals and preferences while the patient is able to participate in a meaning-ful way.

Dementia

In patients with dementia, maintaining function, facilitating independence, and ensuring quality of life remain key management goals, although they may appear very different than in patients with MCI. Dementia encompasses a wide spectrum of disease from mild to advanced; furthermore, the progressive nature of dementia requires ongoing reevaluation and adjustment of goals. Caregiver support becomes increasingly important as disease progresses and dependence increases. Continued vigilance and early intervention for problems such as neuropsychiatric symptoms, sleep disturbance, and incontinence can help maintain the quality of life for both patients and caregivers.

Although early attention to these issues may delay institutionalization, nursing home admission is expected for 75% of those with dementia by age 80 years, compared with just 4% of the general population.[23] Advance care planning and addressing end-of-life wishes increasingly fall to the caregiver as the patient loses capacity to make these decisions, emphasizing the importance of confronting these issues as early as possible in patients with any degree of cognitive impairment. Helping patients and caregivers accept the diagnosis of a terminal illness, and introducing the role of palliative care and hospice are also important management goals for patients with dementia (see later discussion). A summary of management goals at various stages is provided in **Table 3**.

Nonpharmacologic Strategies

Subjective cognitive impairment and mild cognitive impairment

To date, no nonpharmacologic interventions have been shown to prevent further decline in patients with either subjective cognitive impairment or MCI. Subjective cognitive impairment is a relatively new construct, and few strategies to delay progres-sion have been studied. Investigations into nonpharmacologic strategies for MCI have been complicated by the heterogeneity and instability of this diagnosis. Two promising strategies that have been studied in MCI are exercise[24–27] and cognitive training,[26–33] although the quality and quantity of evidence is limited, and more rigorous controlled trials in well-defined populations are needed. Because both exercise and cognitive training are associated with few, if any, risks and may have beneficial effects on cogni-tion, patients with subjective cognitive impairment or MCI should be advised to adopt both of these activities as part of an overall healthy lifestyle. Both the US Centers for Disease Control and Prevention[34] and the National Institute on Aging[34] have guide-lines for physical activity in older adults and materials that can be used to help patients initiate and maintain a regular exercise program. Patients should be encouraged to

Table 3
Management goals for elderly patients with cognitive complaints

Management Goal	Subjective Cognitive Complaint	MCI	Dementia
Maintain independence and quality of life	←———————————————→		
Optimize management of comorbidities	←———————————————→		
Treat vascular risk factors	←———————————————→		
Eliminate/minimize medications affecting cognitive function	←———————————————→		
Promote physical and mental health	←———————————————→		
Advance care planning	←———————————————→		
Ongoing monitoring for progression	←———————————————→		
Acceptance and adjusting expectations		←——————————→	
Referral to support organization		←——————————→	
Partnership with patient and caregiver		←——————————→	
Caregiver support			←——→
Meeting goals/preferences for end-of-life care			←——→

Abbreviation: MCI, mild cognitive impairment.

engage in enjoyable, cognitively stimulating activities. There are no compelling data to support any specific program or activity; patients should pursue activities that match their interests and abilities.

Dementia

Numerous nonpharmacologic interventions targeting patients with dementia, their caregivers, or the patient-caregiver dyad have been investigated (**Box 1**). To date, high-quality evidence for any strategy is lacking, as most studies tend to be small, heterogeneous with respect to populations, interventions, and outcomes, and/or of poor quality.

One of the more promising nonpharmacologic interventions is exercise. Possible mechanisms by which exercise may improve or maintain cognitive function include improving central adiposity and insulin resistance,[35–37] decreasing oxidative stress and low-grade inflammation,[38] improving vascular function,[39] and increasing cerebral blood flow.[40] Combined with the established benefits of exercise on multiple chronic illnesses and lack of side effects when properly performed, exercise presents an extremely attractive potential therapy for dementia. Epidemiologic evidence strongly supports a beneficial effect of higher levels of physical activity on cognitive function and the risk of dementia,[41] but results from prospective randomized controlled trials (RCTs) have been mixed. A recent review of 6 good-quality RCTs found that all reported significant positive results on functional outcomes.[42] The most recent Cochrane review concluded that exercise interventions may have positive effects on cognitive function and activities of daily living, but emphasized that significant heterogeneity among studies requires cautious interpretation of results.[43] In addition, research to determine the optimal type, duration, and intensity of exercise for patients with dementia is needed. As with MCI, regular physical activity should be recommended for all patients with dementia.

Cognitive stimulation uses enjoyable activities to engage memory and concentration in a social setting. Two of the larger studies using this approach reported improvements in cognitive function[44,45] and quality of life,[44] but not in functional status, mood, or behavioral symptoms. Cognitive training or rehabilitation has also received considerable attention, resulting in a burgeoning commercial industry promoting "brain training" programs to enhance or maintain cognitive function. To date, studies of these

---

Box 1
Nonpharmacologic interventions investigated in dementia

- Exercise[43]
- Cognitive stimulation[124]
- Cognitive training/rehabilitation[46]
- Reminiscence therapy[128,129]
- Bright light therapy[131]
- Massage/touch therapy[133]
- Music therapy[122,123]
- Aromatherapy[125,126]
- Transcutaneous electrical nerve stimulation (TENS)[127]
- Respite care for caregivers[130]
- Cognitive reframing for caregivers[132]

interventions in patients with mild to moderate dementia have not provided strong evidence of benefit on cognition, function, or mood,[46] and patients and caregivers should be cautioned against expensive programs that promise to prevent or reverse dementia. Most studies are of low to moderate quality, and have been small and of short duration. Outcomes such as trajectory of decline or time to institutionalization have not been studied. However, given the risk/benefit ratio and the lack of effective treatments for dementia, patients should be encouraged to participate in enjoyable, cognitively stimulating activities appropriate for their interests and level of impairment.

Neuropsychiatric symptoms

Managing neuropsychiatric symptoms in patients with dementia can be extremely challenging and distressing for caregivers, and often serve as the trigger for institutionalization. These symptoms may reflect unmet needs (eg, pain, constipation, urinary tract infection), unintentional reinforcement of behaviors (eg, repetitive questioning or yelling to receive attention), or lack of fit between the environment and the patient's abilities (eg, excess stimulation or distraction).[47] Nonpharmacologic approaches to managing these symptoms are strongly preferred because of the limited benefits and substantial risks of pharmacologic therapies (discussed in the next section). General strategies for managing behavioral symptoms are described in **Table 4**.[48–50]

Table 4
Nonpharmacologic strategies for neuropsychiatric symptoms in dementia

Symptom	Strategies
Depression/apathy	Introduce/encourage enjoyable activities Modify activities patient has enjoyed in the past to fit current level of function to avoid frustration Consider repetitive activities (eg, folding laundry, sorting papers) Introduce/encourage social activities, outings Address caregiver depression
Agitation	Identify and avoid triggers Maintain structured daily routines Stay calm; avoid arguing, reasoning Redirect and distract
Wandering	Provide labels or visual cues (eg, arrows to bathroom, bedroom, stop signs) Disguise exits Provide supervision (eg, family, paid caregivers, adult day programs) Introduce/encourage enjoyable activities Develop a safety plan (eg, "Safe Return" program)
Hallucinations/delusions	If not disturbing or frightening, allow patient their experience of the truth; avoid reasoning or attempting to correct patient's perceptions If disturbing or frightening provide calm reassurance, distract and redirect, consider medication
Disorientation	Simplify environment, reduce clutter, noise Provide visual cues and reminders Provide verbal prompts Identify self and others
Sleep disturbance	Maintain consistent sleep times and routines Avoid daytime napping Reduce/eliminate alcohol and caffeine Reduce/eliminate noise, distractions Consider bright light exposure

Specific interventions should match the patient's needs and abilities, which will change as the disease progresses. Successful implementation of these strategies is more likely with a team approach involving the patient, caregiver(s), and multiple health professionals. This approach can be time consuming and labor intensive, and is not well supported by current reimbursement systems, presenting significant barriers to more widespread use.

Pharmacologic Strategies

Options for pharmacologic treatment of cognitive impairment are few and limited to dementia. There are no approved pharmacologic therapies for MCI, and no studies have yet been conducted in patients with subjective cognitive impairment. Despite 30 years of drug development efforts, there are only 4 medications in 2 drug classes approved by the Food and Drug Administration that are available for the treatment of dementia (**Table 5**). These drugs are approved only for AD with the exception of rivastigmine, which is also approved for Parkinson disease dementia (PDD).

Cholinesterase inhibitors

The cholinesterase inhibitors (ChEIs) prevent the enzymatic breakdown of the neurotransmitter acetylcholine in the synaptic cleft. Cholinergic transmission is thought to be crucial for attention and memory, in addition to neuronal plasticity, and as early as 1976 severe cortical cholinergic loss was noted in AD patients.[51,52] Although enthusiasm for ChEIs waned as attempts at disease-modifying amyloid-based therapies began to dominate research efforts, these drugs remain the mainstay of pharmacologic therapy for dementia.

The effectiveness of the ChEIs has been summarized in several systematic reviews and meta-analyses.[53–55] The data support modest benefits in stabilizing or slowing cognitive decline, behavior, and function, but the clinical significance of the changes is uncertain. Comparisons between ChEIs suggest that all 3 drugs are similarly effective.

ChEIs have not been as well studied in dementias other than AD. Small improvements in cognition, behavior, and function in PDD have been reported, but the clinical benefit in LBD is not clear.[56] Donepezil has been studied in patients with probable mild to moderate vascular dementia, with small improvements in cognition and function compared with placebo[57]; evidence for benefit with rivastigmine[58] and galantamine[59] are less certain. ChEIs should not be used in the treatment of frontotemporal dementia, in which no cholinergic deficit has been demonstrated.[60] Although one small, open-label study showed improvement in some behavioral symptoms with rivastigmine,[61] other studies of ChEIs in frontotemporal dementia showed no benefit[62] and potential worsening[63] of symptoms.

Side effects of ChEIs are related to increases in cholinergic activity and most commonly include nausea, vomiting, and diarrhea, which can often be minimized with dose titration over 4 to 6 weeks. In addition, augmentation of parasympathetic activity has been associated with an increased risk of syncope,[64,65] hospitalization for bradycardia,[66] pacemaker insertion,[64] and hip fracture.[64] In addition to awareness of potential side effects, it is important for patients and caregivers to understand that although ChEIs may provide some symptomatic benefits, they do not change the underlying course of the disease. There is no clear consensus on the appropriate duration of treatment with ChEIs. Recent guidelines from the American Geriatrics Society as part of the "Choosing Wisely" Campaign recommended a trial of 12 weeks if the medication is tolerated, as any benefit is likely to be observed by then.[67] Because "improvement" may manifest as stability or a slower rate of decline, and bedside

Table 5
Approved pharmacologic treatments for dementia

Drug	Year Approved	FDA-Labeled Indications	Dosing		Route	Frequency
			Initial	Maintenance		
Cholinesterase Inhibitors						
Donepezil	1996	AD, all stages	5 mg	10 or 23 mg	Oral	Daily
Galantamine-IR	2000	AD, mild to moderate	4 mg	8–12 mg	Oral	BID
Galantamine-ER	2004	AD, mild to moderate	8 mg	16–24 mg	Oral	Daily
Rivastigmine	2001	AD, mild to moderate PDD, mild to moderate	1.5 mg	6 mg	Oral	BID
Rivastigmine patch	2007	AD, all stages[a] PDD, mild to moderate	4.6 mg/24 h	9.5–13.3 mg/24 h	Transdermal	Daily
NDMA Receptor Antagonists						
Memantine	2003	AD, moderate to severe	5 mg	10 mg	Oral	BID
Memantine-ER	2010	AD, moderate to severe	7 mg	28 mg	Oral	Daily

Abbreviations: AD, Alzheimer disease; BID, twice daily; ER, extended release; FDA, Food and Drug Administration; IR, immediate release; NMDA, *N*-methyl-D-aspartate; PDD, Parkinson disease dementia.

[a] High-dose patch (13.3 mg/24 h) approved for severe dementia in 2013.

cognitive assessments are unlikely to show significant change, the decision to continue the medication often depends on the patient and caregivers' perceptions of benefit. If a clinically significant decline is observed after stopping a ChEI, therapy can be restarted. Such treatment gaps do not seem to increase the risk of institution-alization or mortality.[68]

Memantine

The second class of drugs approved for the treatment of dementia is the *N*-methyl-ᴅ-aspartate (NMDA) receptor antagonist memantine. Excessive stimulation of the NMDA receptor by the excitatory neurotransmitter glutamate may result in neuronal excito-toxicity. Memantine is purported to prevent pathologic activation of the NMDA recep-tor via low to moderate affinity binding, thereby providing neuroprotection. Memantine is approved only for moderate to severe AD, with small benefits on cognition, behavior, and function demonstrated with 6 months of treatment in several trials.[69] Memantine does not seem to be effective in mild AD, although its use in this population is common.[70] Memantine is typically well tolerated.

Data supporting the use of memantine in dementia other than AD are mixed. There is some evidence of benefit in patients with vascular dementia,[71,72] but studies in PDD and LBD are inconsistent.[73,74] The few studies conducted to date have not supported a role for memantine in frontotemporal dementia.[75,76]

Combination therapy with ChEI and memantine is appealing given the different mechanisms of action of these drugs, but studies to date have not clearly supported this approach.[77–79] Hopes that ChEIs or memantine would prevent further cognitive or functional decline in MCI have not been realized. One study reported a decreased rate of conversion from MCI to AD with donepezil compared with placebo at 12 months, but by 36 months the conversion rates were not different.[80] Despite the lack of evi-dence, ChEIs and memantine are frequently used in patients with MCI[81]; availability of generic forms of most of these drugs has also likely tilted the cost-benefit calcula-tion toward more widespread use.

In summary, a trial of a ChEI or, in patients with moderate to severe dementia, mem-antine, is recommended in patients without contraindications to the medications after discussion of reasonable expectations of symptomatic benefit and potential side ef-fects. If there is no perceived benefit after at least 12 weeks of therapy, these medica-tions should be discontinued.

Supplements and medical foods

There is no evidence to date that any dietary supplement is effective in delaying or pre-venting cognitive decline.[82] Commonly used supplements for cognitive complaints include gingko biloba, ginseng, B vitamins, vitamin E, omega-3 fatty acids, and phos-pholipids. Many of these supplements have potential adverse effects and drug inter-actions,[83] yet patients often do not inform their health care providers about their use of these supplements unless specifically queried.

Among supplements, the antioxidant vitamin E has been studied most extensively in clinical trials for potential cognitive benefits. Although a positive association between vitamin E and cognitive function has been reported,[84] controlled trials have not convincingly demonstrated benefit. Two trials have reported that vitamin E treatment slowed progression of dementia compared with placebo (measured as decline in functional status, institutionalization, or development of severe dementia or death),[85,86] but no benefit on secondary cognitive outcomes. In addition, both studies had methodological and/or statistical limitations that limit interpretation of results.

As preventive therapy, vitamin E did not delay progression to dementia over 3 years in patients with MCI.[80] Furthermore, concerns about the adverse effects[87,88] and possible increased mortality with vitamin E supplementation[89] have dampened enthusiasm for its use.

Medical foods are intended for "the specific dietary management of a disease or condition for which distinctive nutritional requirements, based on recognized scientific principles, are established by medical evaluation."[90] AC-1202 (Axona) is the only medical food currently available for AD. AC-1202 is a medium-chain triglyceride that is metabolized into ketone bodies, which can be used as an alternative to glucose as an energy source for neurons. In a 90-day RCT of 152 participants with mild to moderate AD, AC-1202 did not improve cognition compared with placebo, although a significant benefit was found in *APOE-ε4*–negative participants.[91]

Pharmacologic treatment of neuropsychiatric symptoms in dementia

The off-label use of antipsychotics for neuropsychiatric symptoms in dementia is common, with an estimated 20% to 30% of patients receiving these medications.[92] Data for the efficacy of antipsychotics are limited, and suggest that the clinical benefits are modest at best.[93–95] Furthermore, these small benefits may be offset by adverse effects and harms. Both typical and atypical antipsychotics are associated with extrapyramidal symptoms, sedation, confusion, and falls. Because patients with LBD are particularly sensitive to these agents, consultation with a specialist (eg, neurologist, geriatric psychiatrist) is recommended.

In addition to adverse effects, both typical and atypical antipsychotic medications are associated with increased mortality.[96–98] Given their limited, uncertain benefits and potential for serious harm, antipsychotics should be reserved for those cases whereby nonpharmacologic strategies have failed and the patient poses a serious threat to himself/herself or others.[99] If started, a risk-benefit discussion with the caregiver should be performed and documented, and frequent review and attempts to withdraw the medications are recommended. Limited data suggest that these agents may be safely withdrawn in patients with dementia without risk of relapse.[100]

Comorbid depression should be considered as a contributor to behavioral disturbance in patients with dementia. Depression may be difficult to diagnose in this population, and geriatric or geriatric psychiatry consultation should be considered if available. There is no strong evidence for the benefit of selective serotonin reuptake inhibitors (SSRIs) in the treatment of depression in patients with dementia,[93,101] and potential adverse effects including hyponatremia, QT prolongation, and falls must be considered. However, SSRIs may be beneficial in individual patients and are recommended by some experts.

Pharmacologic treatment of sleep disturbances is generally avoided in patients with dementia, as this population is even more vulnerable to the negative side effects of sedative-hypnotics than older adults in general. One exception is melatonin, which seems to be well tolerated, although studies in patients with dementia and sleep disturbance have had mixed results.[102–104] Additional data suggest that melatonin may also have a positive effect on nonsleep behavioral disturbances in dementia.[105] Trazodone or mirtazapine are sometimes used, but have not been well studied in patients with dementia. Owing to the risk of adverse events, benzodiazepine receptor agonists, benzodiazepines, and sedating antipsychotics should only be used when all other options have been exhausted and with a risk-benefit discussion with caregivers, as these agents can convey a significant risk of delirium, oversedation, and falls.

Evaluation, Adjustment, and Recurrence

Ongoing evaluation of cognitive status and review of management goals should be incorporated into regular medical visits for patients with any cognitive complaint or impairment. Although some patients may be followed by a neurologist, day-to-day management in the context of the patient's other medical conditions will generally fall to the primary care provider. The primary care provider has a critical role in coordinating care among multiple disciplines such as physical, occupational, and speech therapy, nutrition, social work, and pharmacy. The primary care provider should also keep apprised of care the patient is receiving from any specialists, especially with respect to medications prescribed that may affect cognition, and ensure that the plan of care is consistent with the patient's and family members' goals.

As the disease inevitably advances, the question of discontinuing medications frequently arises. These decisions should be guided by the patient's goals of care, but it is often appropriate to reduce or discontinue medications that are not providing symptomatic benefits, and de-escalate treatment of conditions such as hypertension and diabetes. It may be appropriate to taper and discontinue ChEIs when patients reach an advanced stage of dementia, as benefits are unlikely to be realized. Although memantine is approved for use in severe dementia, the benefits in very advanced stages are uncertain. As noted earlier, the medications can be restarted if a significant decline is noted in relation to stopping.

End-of-life care

Providing quality end-of-life care in patients with cognitive impairment poses special challenges that increase with the degree of impairment, thus the importance of early advance care planning cannot be overstated. Palliative care is appropriate for all patients with a diagnosis of dementia, given the terminal nature of this disease and its associated physical and psychological symptoms. Difficulty with swallowing and walking, weakness, incontinence, and sleep disruption often occur as disease progresses. Symptoms related to comorbid conditions such as pain and dyspnea may also be present. One of the major challenges in providing palliative care to patients with cognitive impairment is communication, as patients may be unable to describe their symptoms or whether interventions are effective.

Hospice care has the potential to provide significant benefits for patients with dementia, including better quality of life[106,107] and increased caregiver and family satisfaction.[108] Compared with nonhospice dementia patients, those enrolled in hospice are more likely to die in their location of choice[108] and to have a better overall dying experience.[106,107] Use of hospice for dementia patients has been steadily increasing; an analysis of Medicare data reported that the proportion of patients with dementia enrolled in hospice at the time of death increased from 19.5% in 2000 to 48.5% in 2009.[109] Countering this encouraging trend, however, were increases in intensive care unit utilization and mechanical ventilation within the last 30 days of life, an increase in the proportion of patients with dementia who transitioned between sites of care in the last 3 days of life, and in late hospice referrals (enrollment within 3 days of death). Alarmingly, a recent study of greater than 4700 discharges from hospice care found that patients with dementia were significantly more likely than patients with other diagnoses to have received tube feeding,[110] even though ample evidence suggests that tube feeding provides no morbidity or mortality benefit in this population.[111] These data suggest that despite increased hospice utilization in patients with dementia, significant barriers to providing high-quality end-of-life care for this population remain.

Several characteristics of dementia may act as potential barriers to improving end-of-life care. Despite heightened awareness of dementia, both the public and professional communities have difficulty recognizing dementia as a terminal disease. Indeed, one of the most common questions about dementia is what patients with dementia actually die from; the terminal event (eg, pneumonia, urinary tract infection), rather than the dementia, is often considered the proximate cause of death.[112] Acceptance of dementia as a terminal disease is further complicated by the trajectory of death and the considerable prognostic uncertainty, which has been cited as the primary barrier to hospice enrollment.[113] Current Medicare hospice eligibility requirements are based on assessment of functional status and the occurrence of specific medical conditions.[114] These somewhat rigid criteria have been shown to be poor predictors of life expectancy in dementia,[115–117] which may explain in part the high hospice disenrollment rates in patients with this diagnosis.[110] The lack of fit between the current hospice model and the nature of dementia has led some experts to suggest a shift in focus from prognosis to early palliative care guided by a preference for comfort.[110] Choosing to forgo life-prolonging interventions in dementia can be extremely challenging for both caregivers and health care providers, especially when the treatment seems relatively nonburdensome. For example, a decision not to provide intravenous fluids and antibiotic treatment for a urinary tract infection to a patient with advanced dementia may be fraught with guilt and uncertainty, given that withholding this simple intervention may be perceived as hastening the patient's death.

The primary care provider has an essential role in end-of-life care for patients with dementia. Establishing and frequently revisiting goals of care and providing information on risks and benefits of specific treatments can help prevent burdensome interventions and transitions at the end of life. Ensuring the timely introduction of palliative care and hospice services can provide a better quality of life and better dying experience for both patients and their caregivers, although challenges to delivering these effectively and efficiently within the current system remain.

FUTURE CONSIDERATIONS AND SUMMARY

As the population of older adults continues to increase, health care providers in virtually all specialties will be caring for growing numbers of patients with cognitive impairment and dementia, most commonly AD. At present, our ability to diagnose and treat conditions along the spectrum of cognitive impairment is disappointingly limited. Approved medications provide modest symptomatic benefits in some patients, but do not affect the underlying course of the disease. Nonpharmacologic approaches form the cornerstone of management, with a focus on maintaining function and independence, and providing caregiver support.

To date, efforts to develop effective preventive and treatment strategies for dementia, particularly AD, have been hampered by the long time lag between neurologic damage and the onset of clinical disease. Although significant progress has been made in the development of biomarkers to diagnose AD both earlier and with more certainty, the heterogeneity of AD will likely require a multifaceted approach to prevention and treatment that addresses the varying risk factors that may contribute to the development and progression of cognitive impairment in different populations.

REFERENCES

1. Lin JS, O'Connor E, Rossom RC, et al. Screening for cognitive impairment in older adults: a systematic review for the U.S. Preventive Services Task Force. Ann Intern Med 2013;159(9):601–12.

Cognitive Complaints in the Elderly   **329**

2. Cordell CB, Borson S, Boustani M, et al. Alzheimer's Association recommendations for operationalizing the detection of cognitive impairment during the Medicare annual wellness visit in a primary care setting. Alzheimers Dement 2013; 9(2):141–50.
3. Reisberg B, Gauthier S. Current evidence for subjective cognitive impairment (SCI) as the pre-mild cognitive impairment (MCI) stage of subsequently manifest Alzheimer's disease. Int Psychogeriatr 2008;20(1):1–16.
4. Reisberg B, Shulman MB, Torossian C, et al. Outcome over seven years of healthy adults with and without subjective cognitive impairment. Alzheimers Dement 2010;6(1):11–24.
5. Petersen RC. Mild cognitive impairment as a diagnostic entity. J Intern Med 2004;256(3):183–94.
6. Boyle PA, Wilson RS, Aggarwal NT, et al. Mild cognitive impairment: risk of Alzheimer disease and rate of cognitive decline. Neurology 2006;67(3):441–5.
7. Petersen RC, Smith GE, Waring SC, et al. Mild cognitive impairment: clinical characterization and outcome. Arch Neurol 1999;56(3):303–8.
8. Larrieu S, Letenneur L, Orgogozo JM, et al. Incidence and outcome of mild cognitive impairment in a population-based prospective cohort. Neurology 2002;59(10):1594–9.
9. Ritchie K, Artero S, Touchon J. Classification criteria for mild cognitive impairment: a population-based validation study. Neurology 2001;56(1):37–42.
10. Ganguli M, Dodge HH, Shen C, et al. Mild cognitive impairment, amnestic type: an epidemiologic study. Neurology 2004;63(1):115–21.
11. Albert MS, DeKosky ST, Dickson D, et al. The diagnosis of mild cognitive impairment due to Alzheimer's disease: recommendations from the National Institute on Aging-Alzheimer's Association workgroups on diagnostic guidelines for Alzheimer's disease. Alzheimers Dement 2011;7(3):270–9.
12. McKhann GM, Knopman DS, Chertkow H, et al. The diagnosis of dementia due to Alzheimer's disease: recommendations from the National Institute on Aging-Alzheimer's Association workgroups on diagnostic guidelines for Alzheimer's disease. Alzheimers Dement 2011;7(3):263–9.
13. Gorelick PB, Scuteri A, Black SE, et al. Vascular contributions to cognitive impairment and dementia: a statement for healthcare professionals from the American Heart Association/American Stroke Association. Stroke 2011;42(9): 2672–713.
14. MacLullich AM, Beaglehole A, Hall RJ, et al. Delirium and long-term cognitive impairment. Int Rev Psychiatry 2009;21(1):30–42.
15. Ballard CG, Gauthier S, Cummings JL, et al. Management of agitation and aggression associated with Alzheimer disease. Nat Rev Neurol 2009;5(5):245–55.
16. Savva GM, Wharton SB, Ince PG, et al. Age, neuropathology, and dementia. N Engl J Med 2009;360(22):2302–9.
17. Hardy J, Selkoe DJ. The amyloid hypothesis of Alzheimer's disease: progress and problems on the road to therapeutics. Science 2002;297(5580):353–6.
18. Querfurth HW, LaFerla FM. Alzheimer's disease. N Engl J Med 2010;362(4): 329–44.
19. Dickson DW. Neuropathology of non-Alzheimer degenerative disorders. Int J Clin Exp Pathol 2009;3(1):1–23.
20. Larson EB, Yaffe K, Langa KM. New insights into the dementia epidemic. N Engl J Med 2013;369(24):2275–7.
21. Knopman DS, DeKosky ST, Cummings JL, et al. Practice parameter: diagnosis of dementia (an evidence-based review). Report of the Quality Standards

Subcommittee of the American Academy of Neurology. Neurology 2001;56(9): 1143–53.

22. Duthie EH, Katz PR, Malone ML. Practice of geriatrics. 4th edition. Philadelphia: Saunders Elsevier; 2007.

23. Arrighi HM, Neumann PJ, Lieberburg IM, et al. Lethality of Alzheimer disease and its impact on nursing home placement. Alzheimer Dis Assoc Disord 2010;24(1):90–5.

24. Heyn P, Abreu BC, Ottenbacher KJ. The effects of exercise training on elderly persons with cognitive impairment and dementia: a meta-analysis. Arch Phys Med Rehabil 2004;85(10):1694–704.

25. Lautenschlager NT, Cox KL, Flicker L, et al. Effect of physical activity on cognitive function in older adults at risk for Alzheimer disease: a randomized trial. JAMA 2008;300(9):1027–37.

26. Teixeira CV, Gobbi LT, Corazza DI, et al. Non-pharmacological interventions on cognitive functions in older people with mild cognitive impairment (MCI). Arch Gerontol Geriatr 2012;54(1):175–80.

27. Wang C, Yu JT, Wang HF, et al. Non-pharmacological interventions for patients with mild cognitive impairment: a meta-analysis of randomized controlled trials of cognition-based and exercise interventions. J Alzheimers Dis 2014;42:663–78.

28. Martin M, Clare L, Altgassen AM, et al. Cognition-based interventions for healthy older people and people with mild cognitive impairment. Cochrane Database Syst Rev 2011;(1):CD006220.

29. Olchik MR, Farina J, Steibel N, et al. Memory training (MT) in mild cognitive impairment (MCI) generates change in cognitive performance. Arch Gerontol Geriatr 2013;56(3):442–7.

30. Gagnon LG, Belleville S. Training of attentional control in mild cognitive impairment with executive deficits: results from a double-blind randomised controlled study. Neuropsychol Rehabil 2012;22(6):809–35.

31. Li H, Li J, Li N, et al. Cognitive intervention for persons with mild cognitive impairment: a meta-analysis. Ageing Res Rev 2011;10(2):285–96.

32. Belleville S, Gilbert B, Fontaine F, et al. Improvement of episodic memory in persons with mild cognitive impairment and healthy older adults: evidence from a cognitive intervention program. Dement Geriatr Cogn Disord 2006;22(5–6):486–99.

33. Jean L, Bergeron ME, Thivierge S, et al. Cognitive intervention programs for individuals with mild cognitive impairment: systematic review of the literature. Am J Geriatr Psychiatry 2010;18(4):281–96.

34. Available at: http://go4life.nia.nih.gov/. Accessed September 10, 2014.

35. Baker LD, Frank LL, Foster-Schubert K, et al. Aerobic exercise improves cognition for older adults with glucose intolerance, a risk factor for Alzheimer's disease. J Alzheimers Dis 2010;22(2):569–79.

36. Ryan AS. Insulin resistance with aging: effects of diet and exercise. Sports Med 2000;30(5):327–46.

37. Goodpaster BH, Kelley DE, Wing RR, et al. Effects of weight loss on regional fat distribution and insulin sensitivity in obesity. Diabetes 1999;48(4):839–47.

38. Teixeira-Lemos E, Nunes S, Teixeira F, et al. Regular physical exercise training assists in preventing type 2 diabetes development: focus on its antioxidant and anti-inflammatory properties. Cardiovasc Diabetol 2011;10:12.

39. Fujita S, Rasmussen BB, Cadenas JG, et al. Aerobic exercise overcomes the age-related insulin resistance of muscle protein metabolism by improving endothelial function and Akt/mammalian target of rapamycin signaling. Diabetes 2007;56(6):1615–22.

40. Bolduc V, Thorin-Trescases N, Thorin E. Endothelium-dependent control of cerebrovascular functions through age: exercise for healthy cerebrovascular aging. Am J Physiol Heart Circ Physiol 2013;305(5):H620–33.
41. Rolland Y, Abellan van Kan G, Vellas B. Healthy brain aging: role of exercise and physical activity. Clin Geriatr Med 2010;26(1):75–87.
42. McLaren AN, Lamantia MA, Callahan CM. Systematic review of non-pharmacologic interventions to delay functional decline in community-dwelling patients with dementia. Aging Ment Health 2013;17(6):655–66.
43. Forbes D, Thiessen EJ, Blake CM, et al. Exercise programs for people with dementia. Cochrane Database Syst Rev 2013;(12):CD006489.
44. Spector A, Thorgrimsen L, Woods B, et al. Efficacy of an evidence-based cognitive stimulation therapy programme for people with dementia: randomised controlled trial. Br J Psychiatry 2003;183:248–54.
45. Onder G, Zanetti O, Giacobini E, et al. Reality orientation therapy combined with cholinesterase inhibitors in Alzheimer's disease: randomised controlled trial. Br J Psychiatry 2005;187:450–5.
46. Bahar-Fuchs A, Clare L, Woods B. Cognitive training and cognitive rehabilitation for mild to moderate Alzheimer's disease and vascular dementia. Cochrane Database Syst Rev 2013;(6):CD003260.
47. Cohen-Mansfield J. Nonpharmacologic interventions for inappropriate behaviors in dementia: a review, summary, and critique. Am J Geriatr Psychiatry 2001;9(4):361–81.
48. Gitlin LN, Kales HC, Lyketsos CG. Nonpharmacologic management of behavioral symptoms in dementia. JAMA 2012;308(19):2020–9.
49. Sadowsky CH, Galvin JE. Guidelines for the management of cognitive and behavioral problems in dementia. J Am Board Fam Med 2012;25(3): 350–66.
50. Teri L, Logsdon RG, McCurry SM. Nonpharmacologic treatment of behavioral disturbance in dementia. Med Clin North Am 2002;86(3):641–56, viii.
51. Davies P, Maloney AJ. Selective loss of central cholinergic neurons in Alzheimer's disease. Lancet 1976;2(8000):1403.
52. Bowen DM, Smith CB, White P, et al. Neurotransmitter-related enzymes and indices of hypoxia in senile dementia and other abiotrophies. Brain 1976; 99(3):459–96.
53. Birks J. Cholinesterase inhibitors for Alzheimer's disease. Cochrane Database Syst Rev 2006;(1):CD005593.
54. Hansen RA, Gartlehner G, Webb AP, et al. Efficacy and safety of donepezil, galantamine, and rivastigmine for the treatment of Alzheimer's disease: a systematic review and meta-analysis. Clin Interv Aging 2008;3(2):211–25.
55. Tan CC, Yu JT, Wang HF, et al. Efficacy and safety of donepezil, galantamine, rivastigmine, and memantine for the treatment of Alzheimer's disease: a systematic review and meta-analysis. J Alzheimers Dis 2014;41(2):615–31.
56. Rolinski M, Fox C, Maidment I, et al. Cholinesterase inhibitors for dementia with Lewy bodies, Parkinson's disease dementia and cognitive impairment in Parkinson's disease. Cochrane Database Syst Rev 2012;(3):CD006504.
57. Malouf R, Birks J. Donepezil for vascular cognitive impairment. Cochrane Database Syst Rev 2004;(1):CD004395.
58. Birks J, McGuinness B, Craig D. Rivastigmine for vascular cognitive impairment. Cochrane Database Syst Rev 2013;(5):CD004744.
59. Birks J, Craig D. Galantamine for vascular cognitive impairment. Cochrane Database Syst Rev 2013;(4):CD004746.

60. Francis PT, Holmes C, Webster MT, et al. Preliminary neurochemical findings in non-Alzheimer dementia due to lobar atrophy. Dementia 1993;4(3–4): 172–7.

61. Moretti R, Torre P, Antonello RM, et al. Rivastigmine in frontotemporal dementia: an open-label study. Drugs Aging 2004;21(14):931–7.

62. Kertesz A, Morlog D, Light M, et al. Galantamine in frontotemporal dementia and primary progressive aphasia. Dement Geriatr Cogn Disord 2008;25(2): 178–85.

63. Mendez MF, Shapira JS, McMurtray A, et al. Preliminary findings: behavioral worsening on donepezil in patients with frontotemporal dementia. Am J Geriatr Psychiatry 2007;15(1):84–7.

64. Gill SS, Anderson GM, Fischer HD, et al. Syncope and its consequences in patients with dementia receiving cholinesterase inhibitors: a population-based cohort study. Arch Intern Med 2009;169(9):867–73.

65. Kim DH, Brown RT, Ding EL, et al. Dementia medications and risk of falls, syncope, and related adverse events: meta-analysis of randomized controlled trials. J Am Geriatr Soc 2011;59(6):1019–31.

66. Park-Wyllie LY, Mamdani MM, Li P, et al. Cholinesterase inhibitors and hospitalization for bradycardia: a population-based study. PLoS Med 2009;6(9): e1000157.

67. AGS Choosing Wisely Workgroup. American Geriatrics Society identifies another five things that healthcare providers and patients should question. J Am Geriatr Soc 2014;62(5):950–60.

68. Pariente A, Fourrier-Reglat A, Bazin F, et al. Effect of treatment gaps in elderly patients with dementia treated with cholinesterase inhibitors. Neurology 2012; 78(13):957–63.

69. McShane R, Areosa Sastre A, Minakaran N. Memantine for dementia. Cochrane Database Syst Rev 2006;(2):CD003154.

70. Schneider LS, Dagerman KS, Higgins JP, et al. Lack of evidence for the efficacy of memantine in mild Alzheimer disease. Arch Neurol 2011;68(8):991–8.

71. Orgogozo JM, Rigaud AS, Stoffler A, et al. Efficacy and safety of memantine in patients with mild to moderate vascular dementia: a randomized, placebo-controlled trial (MMM 300). Stroke 2002;33(7):1834–9.

72. Wilcock G, Mobius HJ, Stoffler A. A double-blind, placebo-controlled multi-centre study of memantine in mild to moderate vascular dementia (MMM500). Int Clin Psychopharmacol 2002;17(6):297–305.

73. Aarsland D, Ballard C, Walker Z, et al. Memantine in patients with Parkinson's disease dementia or dementia with Lewy bodies: a double-blind, placebo-controlled, multicentre trial. Lancet Neurol 2009;8(7):613–8.

74. Emre M, Tsolaki M, Bonuccelli U, et al. Memantine for patients with Parkinson's disease dementia or dementia with Lewy bodies: a randomised, double-blind, placebo-controlled trial. Lancet Neurol 2010;9(10):969–77.

75. Boxer AL, Lipton AM, Womack K, et al. An open-label study of memantine treatment in 3 subtypes of frontotemporal lobar degeneration. Alzheimer Dis Assoc Disord 2009;23(3):211–7.

76. Diehl-Schmid J, Forstl H, Perneczky R, et al. 6-month, open-label study of memantine in patients with frontotemporal dementia. Int J Geriatr Psychiatry 2008; 23(7):754–9.

77. Tariot PN, Farlow MR, Grossberg GT, et al. Memantine treatment in patients with moderate to severe Alzheimer disease already receiving donepezil: a randomized controlled trial. JAMA 2004;291(3):317–24.

78. Porsteinsson AP, Grossberg GT, Mintzer J, et al. Memantine treatment in patients with mild to moderate Alzheimer's disease already receiving a cholinesterase inhibitor: a randomized, double-blind, placebo-controlled trial. Curr Alzheimer Res 2008;5(1):83–9.
79. Howard R, McShane R, Lindesay J, et al. Donepezil and memantine for moderate-to-severe Alzheimer's disease. N Engl J Med 2012;366(10):893–903.
80. Petersen RC, Thomas RG, Grundman M, et al. Vitamin E and donepezil for the treatment of mild cognitive impairment. N Engl J Med 2005;352(23):2379–88.
81. Cooper C, Li R, Lyketsos C, et al. Treatment for mild cognitive impairment: systematic review. Br J Psychiatry 2013;203(3):255–64.
82. Daviglus ML, Bell CC, Berrettini W, et al. National Institutes of Health State-of-the-Science Conference statement: preventing Alzheimer disease and cognitive decline. Ann Intern Med 2010;153(3):176–81.
83. Ernst E. The risk-benefit profile of commonly used herbal therapies: ginkgo, St. John's wort, ginseng, echinacea, saw palmetto, and kava. Ann Intern Med 2002; 136(1):42–53.
84. Mangialasche F, Xu W, Kivipelto M, et al. Tocopherols and tocotrienols plasma levels are associated with cognitive impairment. Neurobiol Aging 2012;33(10): 2282–90.
85. Dysken MW, Sano M, Asthana S, et al. Effect of vitamin E and memantine on functional decline in Alzheimer disease: the TEAM-AD VA cooperative randomized trial. JAMA 2014;311(1):33–44.
86. Sano M, Ernesto C, Thomas RG, et al. A controlled trial of selegiline, alpha-tocopherol, or both as treatment for Alzheimer's disease. The Alzheimer's Disease Cooperative Study. N Engl J Med 1997;336(17):1216–22.
87. Lonn E, Bosch J, Yusuf S, et al. Effects of long-term vitamin E supplementation on cardiovascular events and cancer: a randomized controlled trial. JAMA 2005;293(11):1338–47.
88. Schurks M, Glynn RJ, Rist PM, et al. Effects of vitamin E on stroke subtypes: meta-analysis of randomised controlled trials. BMJ 2010;341:c5702.
89. Miller ER 3rd, Pastor-Barriuso R, Dalal D, et al. Meta-analysis: high-dosage vitamin E supplementation may increase all-cause mortality. Ann Intern Med 2005;142(1):37–46.
90. U.S. Food and Drug Administration. Medical foods guidance documents & regulatory information. Available at: http://www.fda.gov/food/guidanceregulation/guidancedocumentsregulatoryinformation/medicalfoods/default.htm. Accessed August 4, 2014.
91. Henderson ST, Vogel JL, Barr LJ, et al. Study of the ketogenic agent AC-1202 in mild to moderate Alzheimer's disease: a randomized, double-blind, placebo-controlled, multicenter trial. Nutr Metab 2009;6:31.
92. Schulze J, Glaeske G, van den Bussche H, et al. Prescribing of antipsychotic drugs in patients with dementia: a comparison with age-matched and sex-matched non-demented controls. Pharmacoepidemiol Drug Saf 2013;22(12):1308–16.
93. Sink KM, Holden KF, Yaffe K. Pharmacological treatment of neuropsychiatric symptoms of dementia: a review of the evidence. JAMA 2005;293(5):596–608.
94. Schneider LS, Tariot PN, Dagerman KS, et al. Effectiveness of atypical antipsychotic drugs in patients with Alzheimer's disease. N Engl J Med 2006;355(15): 1525–38.
95. Maher AR, Maglione M, Bagley S, et al. Efficacy and comparative effectiveness of atypical antipsychotic medications for off-label uses in adults: a systematic review and meta-analysis. JAMA 2011;306(12):1359–69.

96. Schneider LS, Dagerman KS, Insel P. Risk of death with atypical antipsychotic drug treatment for dementia: meta-analysis of randomized placebo-controlled trials. JAMA 2005;294(15):1934–43.

97. Gill SS, Bronskill SE, Normand SL, et al. Antipsychotic drug use and mortality in older adults with dementia. Ann Intern Med 2007;146(11):775–86.

98. Schneeweiss S, Setoguchi S, Brookhart A, et al. Risk of death associated with the use of conventional versus atypical antipsychotic drugs among elderly patients. CMAJ 2007;176(5):627–32.

99. AGS Choosing Wisely Workgroup. American Geriatrics Society identifies five things that healthcare providers and patients should question. J Am Geriatr Soc 2013;61(4):622–31.

100. Declercq T, Petrovic M, Azermai M, et al. Withdrawal versus continuation of chronic antipsychotic drugs for behavioural and psychological symptoms in older people with dementia. Cochrane Database Syst Rev 2013;(3):CD007726.

101. Sepehry AA, Lee PE, Hsiung GY, et al. Effect of selective serotonin reuptake inhibitors in Alzheimer's disease with comorbid depression: a meta-analysis of depression and cognitive outcomes. Drugs Aging 2012;29(10):793–806.

102. Serfaty M, Kennell-Webb S, Warner J, et al. Double blind randomised placebo controlled trial of low dose melatonin for sleep disorders in dementia. Int J Geriatr Psychiatry 2002;17(12):1120–7.

103. Gehrman PR, Connor DJ, Martin JL, et al. Melatonin fails to improve sleep or agitation in double-blind randomized placebo-controlled trial of institutionalized patients with Alzheimer disease. Am J Geriatr Psychiatry 2009;17(2):166–9.

104. Singer C, Tractenberg RE, Kaye J, et al. A multicenter, placebo-controlled trial of melatonin for sleep disturbance in Alzheimer's disease. Sleep 2003;26(7):893–901.

105. Jansen SL, Forbes DA, Duncan V, et al. Melatonin for cognitive impairment. Cochrane Database Syst Rev 2006;(1):CD003802.

106. Kiely DK, Givens JL, Shaffer ML, et al. Hospice use and outcomes in nursing home residents with advanced dementia. J Am Geriatr Soc 2010;58(12):2284–91.

107. Teno JM, Gozalo PL, Lee IC, et al. Does hospice improve quality of care for persons dying from dementia? J Am Geriatr Soc 2011;59(8):1531–6.

108. Shega JW, Hougham GW, Stocking CB, et al. Patients dying with dementia: experience at the end of life and impact of hospice care. J Pain Symptom Manage 2008;35(5):499–507.

109. Teno JM, Gozalo PL, Bynum JP, et al. Change in end-of-life care for Medicare beneficiaries: site of death, place of care, and health care transitions in 2000, 2005, and 2009. JAMA 2013;309(5):470–7.

110. Albrecht JS, Gruber-Baldini AL, Fromme EK, et al. Quality of hospice care for individuals with dementia. J Am Geriatr Soc 2013;61(7):1060–5.

111. Sampson EL, Candy B, Jones L. Enteral tube feeding for older people with advanced dementia. Cochrane Database Syst Rev 2009;(2):CD007209.

112. Michel JP, Pautex S, Zekry D, et al. End-of-life care of persons with dementia. J Gerontol A Biol Sci Med Sci 2002;57(10):M640–4.

113. Hanrahan P, Luchins DJ. Access to hospice programs in end-stage dementia: a national survey of hospice programs. J Am Geriatr Soc 1995;43(1):56–9.

114. Medical guidelines for determining prognosis in selected non-cancer diseases. The National Hospice Organization. Hosp J 1996;11(2):47–63.

115. Hanrahan P, Raymond M, McGowan E, et al. Criteria for enrolling dementia patients in hospice: a replication. Am J Hosp Palliat Care 1999;16(1):395–400.

116. Schonwetter RS, Han B, Small BJ, et al. Predictors of six-month survival among patients with dementia: an evaluation of hospice Medicare guidelines. Am J Hosp Palliat Care 2003;20(2):105–13.
117. Mitchell SL, Miller SC, Teno JM, et al. Prediction of 6-month survival of nursing home residents with advanced dementia using ADEPT vs hospice eligibility guidelines. JAMA 2010;304(17):1929–35.
118. Folstein MF, Folstein SE, McHugh PR. "Mini-mental state". A practical method for grading the cognitive state of patients for the clinician. J Psychiatr Res 1975; 12(3):189–98.
119. Nasreddine ZS, Phillips NA, Bedirian V, et al. The Montreal Cognitive Assessment, MoCA: a brief screening tool for mild cognitive impairment. J Am Geriatr Soc 2005;53(4):695–9.
120. Tariq SH, Tumosa N, Chibnall JT, et al. Comparison of the Saint Louis University mental status examination and the mini-mental state examination for detecting dementia and mild neurocognitive disorder—a pilot study. Am J Geriatr Psychiatry 2006;14(11):900–10.
121. Borson S, Scanlan J, Brush M, et al. The mini-cog: a cognitive 'vital signs' measure for dementia screening in multi-lingual elderly. Int J Geriatr Psychiatry 2000; 15(11):1021–7.
122. Vink AC, Birks JS, Bruinsma MS, et al. Music therapy for people with dementia. Cochrane Database Syst Rev 2004;(3):CD003477.
123. Ueda T, Suzukamo Y, Sato M, et al. Effects of music therapy on behavioral and psychological symptoms of dementia: a systematic review and meta-analysis. Ageing Res Rev 2013;12(2):628–41.
124. Aguirre E, Woods RT, Spector A, et al. Cognitive stimulation for dementia: a systematic review of the evidence of effectiveness from randomised controlled trials. Ageing Res Rev 2013;12(1):253–62.
125. Thorgrimsen L, Spector A, Wiles A, et al. Aroma therapy for dementia. Cochrane Database Syst Rev 2003;(3):CD003150.
126. Fung JK, Tsang HW, Chung RC. A systematic review of the use of aromatherapy in treatment of behavioral problems in dementia. Geriatr Gerontol Int 2012;12(3): 372–82.
127. Cameron M, Lonergan E, Lee H. Transcutaneous electrical nerve stimulation (TENS) for dementia. Cochrane Database Syst Rev 2003;(3):CD004032.
128. Cotelli M, Manenti R, Zanetti O. Reminiscence therapy in dementia: a review. Maturitas 2012;72(3):203–5.
129. Woods B, Spector A, Jones C, et al. Reminiscence therapy for dementia. Cochrane Database Syst Rev 2005;(2):CD001120.
130. Maayan N, Soares-Weiser K, Lee H. Respite care for people with dementia and their carers. Cochrane Database Syst Rev 2014;(1):CD004396.
131. Forbes D, Culum I, Lischka AR, et al. Light therapy for managing cognitive, sleep, functional, behavioural, or psychiatric disturbances in dementia. Cochrane Database Syst Rev 2009;(4):CD003946.
132. Vernooij-Dassen M, Draskovic I, McCleery J, et al. Cognitive reframing for carers of people with dementia. Cochrane Database Syst Rev 2011;(11):CD005318.
133. Viggo Hansen N, Jorgensen T, Ortenblad L. Massage and touch for dementia. Cochrane Database Syst Rev 2006;(4):CD004989.

Pain Management in the Elderly

Monica Malec, MD[a], Joseph W. Shega, MD[b],*

KEYWORDS

- Pain • Older adult • Pain assessment • Pain management

KEY POINTS

- The critical first step in effective pain management is adequate pain assessment. In the elderly population, this includes an assessment of cognition and sensory impairment.
- An appropriate selection of analgesic entails attention to pain etiology along with physiology of aging and comorbidities.
- Opioids are generally safe and effective analgesics for moderate to severe pain when initiated at low doses and preemptive strategies are incorporated to minimize adverse effects.
- Acetaminophen and topical nonsteroidal anti-inflammatory drugs remain first-line therapies for mild to moderate pain, particularly in osteoarthritis; duloxetine's role in pain management continues to evolve.

INTRODUCTION

Persistent pain is common in older adults and results in substantial morbidity. A recent, nationally representative sample of community-dwelling older adults found that 67% reported pain of moderate or greater intensity over the past 4 weeks.[1,2] The prevalence of pain did not vary significantly between age groups of persons age 60 to 74, 75 to 84, and 85 and older.[1] However, pain prevalence may increase as older adults approach the end of life.[3] Also, older patients often have pain in multiple sites, compounding pain-related suffering and disability.

Pain presence is associated with worse health and those in pain may experience greater functional impairment, falls, depression, decreased appetite, impaired sleep, and social isolation compared with persons not in pain.[4–6] Moreover, the multidimensional impact of pain may leave older adults more vulnerable and less able to effectively respond to physiologic stressors, ultimately contributing to the development of frailty.[7,8] Although pain can be adequately managed in most elderly patients, it remains undertreated, especially in the oldest old, African Americans and other ethnic

[a] Section of Geriatrics and Palliative Medicine, University of Chicago, 5841 S.Maryland avenue, Chicago, IL 60537, USA; [b] VITAS Healthcare, 201 South Biscayne Boulevard Miami, Miami, FL 33131, USA
* Corresponding author. VITAS Healthcare, 2201 Lucien Way #100, Maitland, FL 32751.
E-mail address: jshega@gmail.com

Med Clin N Am 99 (2015) 337–350
http://dx.doi.org/10.1016/j.mcna.2014.11.007
medical.theclinics.com

minorities, and those with cognitive impairment.[9–11] See **Box 1** for patient and provider factors that contribute to the undertreatment of pain in the elderly.

As with any clinical decision, shared decision making is essential to balance the benefits and burdens of pain management interventions, including nonpharmacologic and pharmacologic approaches. Pain management goals should be delineated before the initiation of any therapy with ongoing monitoring of treatment targets and adverse effects over time. Patients and families should be educated that pain can be reduced with currently available treatments; however, the complete elimination of pain is generally not an achievable goal. Also, treatment should generally be targeted at improvements in pain-related disability rather than pain intensity, because improvements in disability are more tangible outcomes among persons with persistent pain. In this review, we provide an overview of pain assessment and management for older adults with management focusing on the initiation and monitoring of commonly used analgesics.

PAIN ASSESSMENT

Adequate pain assessment is the lynchpin of optimal pain management. Given that older adults often suffer with persistent pain for years, clinicians should integrate a comprehensive history and physical examination along with relevant diagnostic tests before developing a treatment plan.[4,12] Family and/or professional caregivers should also be interviewed when possible to corroborate key aspects of the pain history. **Table 1** provides essential components of a standardized pain assessment. Note that an evaluation for sensory and cognitive impairment is an integral part of pain assessment in the elderly patient. For example, hearing loss may make it more difficult for an older adult to interpret and self-report pain on a standard scale.

Pain assessment in persons with cognitive impairment or the nonverbal patient can be particularly challenging and should include an attempt at patient self-report, review of painful conditions, evaluation of pain behaviors, caregiver report of patient's

---

Box 1
Factors leading to undertreatment of pain in elderly patients

Patient factors that may contribute to under treatment of pain

- Pain represents a new or worsening disease process
- Fear of being prescribed an opioid
- Fear of addiction
- Fear of analgesics losing effect and not being effective once pain is severe
- Previous dismissal of pain report by healthcare providers
- Labeled as a weak or difficult patient or a complainer
- Cultural and/or religious beliefs

Provider factors that may contribute to under treatment of pain

- Lack of training in pain assessment and/or management
- Fear of state and federal initiatives scrutinizing physicians who prescribe opioids
- Fear of diversion when an opioid is prescribed
- Fear of opioid-related side effects including increased risk of falls and confusion
- Fear of litigation surrounding any use of opioids

Table 1
Overview of a comprehensive pain assessment

Domain	Components
Pain presence	At rest, with activity
Pain intensity	Now, on an average day, worst pain, lowest level of pain
Pain characteristics	Location, frequency, exacerbating and relieving factors, character, and natural history
Pain physiology	Nociceptive, neuropathic, or mixed
Pain interference with activity and pain-related morbidity	Physical, psychological, spiritual, and social functioning, falls, sleep, appetite, etc
Painful conditions	Osteoarthritis, osteoporosis, previous bone fractures, diabetic neuropathy, post-herpetic neuralgia, myofascial pain syndromes, etc
Pain behavior	Facial expressions, vocalizations, body movements, changes in interpersonal interactions and routines, and mental status changes
Pain treatment	Nonpharmacologic and pharmacologic including injections, surgical interventions, and alternative therapies
Coping style	Distraction, ignoring pain sensations, reinterpreting pain sensations, catastrophizing, praying, and hoping
Sensory	Hearing, vision, and cognition
Proxy report	Professional and family caregiver

experience, and if necessary an empiric analgesic trial.[13] An empiric analgesic trial is an invaluable tool to help distinguish between actual pain and pain perseveration. Persons with cognitive impairment may exhibit pain perseveration (ie, repetitive pain reporting) while not displaying any nonverbal pain behaviors or impaired activity related to pain. A common scenario would be (1) a patient who reports pain and discusses it very frequently during the visit and at home with family, (2) a family caregiver reports the patient consistently talks about pain even though most of the time the patient seems to be comfortable, and (3) few pain behaviors at rest and with activity. When the multifaceted assessment remains inconclusive, an empiric analgesic trial can help to determine whether or not the patient is experiencing significant pain or pain that interferes with function.

GUIDELINES FOR TREATING PAIN

General principles of pain management are well-established and supported by several consensus guidelines, including those from the American Pain Society and the American Geriatrics Society.[4,14] As part of a comprehensive treatment plan, analgesics are often considered to decrease pain intensity and to help improve a patient's well-being.[15] The World Health Organization's 3-step pain ladder, initially developed as an approach for managing cancer-related pain, has been widely accepted and adopted as a guide for selecting analgesics.[4] The underlying premise of the ladder is that pain intensity guides analgesic selection. Step 1 corresponds with mild-intensity pain and includes the use of acetaminophen, nonsteroidal anti-inflammatory drugs (NSAIDs), or both. Step 2 is associated with moderate pain and promotes the use of "mild opioids," generally considered to be combination products, such as acetaminophen or an NSAID added to an opioid or tramadol. Step 3 represents severe pain and suggests the use of "strong opioids," such as morphine, oxycodone, and hydromorphone. Co-analgesics (medications with pain-relieving properties that were not primarily identified as an analgesic but in clinical practice demonstrate either independent or additive analgesic properties) should be considered with each step, with analgesic selection based on the underlying etiology of the pain. For instance, an older adult with moderate to severe pain secondary to post-herpetic neuralgia may be treated first with gabapentin, with the subsequent addition of a combination opioid, such as oxycodone plus acetaminophen.[16]

The adoption of guidelines including opioids for the management of moderate to severe noncancer pain in older adults has led to a dramatic increase in their use over the past decade.[14] This approach is supported by research that indicates opioid use in older adults is associated with decreased pain intensity and improved function.[15] These benefits must be tempered with safety concerns including increased risk of falls, fractures, and hospitalizations.[17,18] A decision to use opioids requires an individualized approach and consideration of drug–drug and drug–disease interactions, as well as benefits and burdens of treatment, including an assessment of risk of diversion and addiction.

PHARMACOLOGIC MANAGEMENT
Acetaminophen

Acetaminophen is the most commonly used analgesic in the United States and is indicated for the management of mild to moderate pain. It does not exhibit significant anti-inflammatory or antiplatelet effects because it does not inhibit thromboxane.[19]

Acetaminophen taken at recommended doses is considered safe. However, inadvertent overdose is possible when patients unknowingly consume multiple acetaminophen-containing products simultaneously; more than 600 over-the-counter products contain acetaminophen for the management of pain, fever, insomnia, and cold and flu symptoms. In fact, nearly one-half of cases of liver failure in the United States are owing to unintentional acetaminophen overdose.[20] The risk of hepatotoxicity led the US Food and Drug Administration (FDA) to lower the recommended maximum daily dose from 4 to 3 g, as well as limit the amount of acetaminophen contained in combination products to 325 mg.[21] Lower doses ($\leq$2 g/d) or avoidance altogether is recommended for patients with underlying liver disease or those who consume 3 or more alcoholic beverages daily. Also, a black box warning was placed on acetaminophen-containing products to highlight the risk of acute liver failure and subsequent need for a liver transplant or death.

Nonsteroidal Anti-inflammatory Drugs

Although studies suggest NSAIDs may be more effective for the management of mild inflammatory pain compared with acetaminophen, the most recent American Geriatric Society guidelines for pain management now state that NSAIDs should be considered "very rarely and with extreme caution."[22] Recommendations against its use, particularly long-term use, stems from its high risk of adverse effects, including on the gastrointestinal (GI), cardiovascular, and renal systems.[23] The risk of GI bleeding with NSAIDs increases with age, dose, and duration of therapy and the presence of GI symptoms, such as dyspepsia and abdominal pain, do not predict who will or will not develop bleeding complications.[24] GI prophylaxis with a proton pump inhibitor with NSAID use may mitigate some of the risk of GI toxicity.[25,26] NSAID cardiovascular effects represent another significant risk to older adults, and include fluid retention, worsening hypertension, congestive heart failure, myocardial infarction, and cerebrovascular accidents. NSAIDs significantly impact the renal system as well contributing to water and sodium retention, decreased renal blood flow, electrolyte imbalances, and acute and chronic renal failure. If an NSAID is being considered for osteoarthritis pain, topical NSAIDs are generally preferred, but a short course of oral NSAIDs may be indicated in the appropriate patient (eg, adequate renal function, no risk factors for GI bleed, and no cardiovascular disease). Common clinical scenarios in which NSAID use may be considered with caution include acute pain, such as a musculoskeletal injury, an episode of acute-on-chronic pain, or someone with arthritis pain unable to tolerate an opioid and not deriving adequate analgesia from scheduled acetaminophen.

Opioids

Opioid medications are recommended and effective for the management of moderate to severe pain and cancer pain in particular. Studies of opioid rotation suggest inter-individual variability in both analgesic response and tolerability.[27] As a result, older adults should be questioned about prior opioid exposure, such as with dental work or after a surgical procedure, along with beneficial or adverse responses to help guide initial opioid selection. Finally, any discussion of opioid therapy in older or younger adults necessitates dialogue and documentation around addiction and diversion, with patients who may be at high risk for addiction being considered for referral to a pain specialist.

Opioid selection in older adults

As in younger adults, important considerations when selecting an initial opioid include response to specific opioids in the past, hepatic and renal function, drug interactions, and available formulations of the agent. Important characteristics of commonly pre-scribed opioids in older persons are outlined in **Table 2**. Side effects of most are similar and are also outlined in the table. Morphine or oxycodone at a dose of 2.5 mg every 6 hours with a plan to follow up within 48 to 72 hours to assess for effi-cacy and adverse effects represents a reasonable starting regimen for patients with moderate to severe pain; details of opioid choice and dosing are discussed elsewhere in this article.

Tramadol, a weak mu-opioid agonist with additional serotonin and norepinephrine reuptake inhibition, is not routinely recommended for older adults with moderate to severe pain, but is commonly used. Importantly, its mu-opioid receptor activity results in a similar side effect profile as other opioids and necessitates similar cautions described herein. In addition, tramadol increases seizure risk, particularly at doses higher than 300 mg/d, the maximum daily dose recommended in an older adult. Also, tramadol may increase suicide risk and should not be prescribed in patients with suicidal ideation. Last, the development of serotonin syndrome may occur with the use of tramadol, particularly with concomitant use of serotonergic drugs. Tramadol should be initiated at 25 mg/d or twice daily and increased in 25-mg increments every 2 to 3 days to an initial goal of 100 mg/d.

Dosing opioids in older adults

Another key component to safe opioid prescribing once appropriate treatment goals have been elucidated and agreed upon and an initial short-acting agent has been selected is the initial dose.[28] The "start low and go slow" approach is essential when dosing opioids. Patients who report severe pain or those who have experienced uncontrolled pain for prolonged periods of time will likely require ongoing titration of opioid therapy to balance pain relief with adverse effects. Frequent reevaluation for analgesia and adverse effects is critical in older persons, should be tailored to the patient's condition, comorbidity, and support system, and may include phone calls, offices visits, or visiting nurse services.

Table 2
Characteristics of commonly prescribed opioids in older adults

Opioid	Potency	WHO Step	Metabolism/Excretion	Common Side Effects	Additional Considerations
Tramadol	Weak	2	Hepatic/renal	Constipation, nausea, appetite loss, drowsiness, dizziness, sweating	Lowers seizure threshold; may precipitate serotonin syndrome in SSRI/SSNRI users
Codeine	Weak	2	Hepatic (CYP2D6)/renal	Constipation, nausea, appetite loss, drowsiness, dizziness, sweating, falls	Variability in metabolism both slow and rapid can cause variability in response
Hydrocodone	Weak	2	Hepatic (CYP2D6)/renal	Anxiety, constipation, dry mouth, headache, nausea	Formulated with acetaminophen, which can increase liver toxicity
Morphine	Strong	3	Hepatic/renal	Constipation, nausea, vomiting, appetite loss	Metabolites accumulate in renal insufficiency
Hydromorphone	Strong	3	Hepatic/renal	Constipation, dizziness, drowsiness, dry mouth	Considered safer in renal insufficiency
Oxycodone	Strong	3	Hepatic (CYP 3A4)/renal	Constipation, dizziness, drowsiness, heartburn, nausea, vomiting	No parenteral preparation available in the United States
Fentanyl[a]	Strong	3	Hepatic/renal	Anxiety, confusion, constipation, headache, indigestion, nausea	Prolonged elimination may occur; structurally different than morphine, thus can be used in morphine allergy
Methadone[b]	Strong	3	Hepatic (≥6 CYP450 enzymes)/fecal	Constipation, dizziness, dry mouth, headache, sweating, nausea	Multiple potential drug interactions; variable PK; associated with QT prolongation; mainly excreted in feces, thus safer in renal failure
Buprenorphine	Strong	3	Hepatic/fecal	Less constipation, nausea, and respiratory depression than other opioids	Can be used safely in the context of renal failure

Abbreviations: CYP, cytochrome pigment; PK, pharmacokinetics; SSNRI, selective serotonin–norepinephrine reuptake inhibitors; SSRI, selective serotonin reuptake inhibitors.
[a] Fentanyl should never be initiated in an opioid-naive patient.
[b] Methadone should be initiated only by experienced practitioners.
Data from Refs.[52-54]

Opioids should be started at 25% to 50% of the recommended dose for adults.[28] For example, a typical oral starting dose of morphine or oxycodone in a younger person is 5 to 10 mg, whereas 2.5 to 5 mg represents an appropriate dose for older persons. As with pain management in other age groups, the dose of the opioid is increased gradually until prespecified treatment targets are reached or unmanageable side effects develop. When a dose increase is considered, it should not be escalated until a steady state has been reached. In general, only 1 analgesic agent should be initiated and titrated at a time to optimally ascertain efficacy and adverse effects.

The time to maximal effect of opioids does not change with aging. The onset of action for oral preparations is approximately 30 minutes (6–10 minutes intravenously and 15 minutes subcutaneously), reaching peak plasma levels (peak effect) in approximately 1 hour and lasting approximately 3 to 4 hours. However, many experts in older adult pain management recommend a longer time interval (usually 6 hours) between doses of short-acting preparations at the initiation of opioid therapy, given the heterogeneity in response found in older persons. A steady state is generally reached at around 4 to 5 half-lives of the drug.

After successful initiation of a short-acting opioid, a sustained-release preparation can be considered to decrease medication complexity. Although sustained-release preparations may improve adherence and patient satisfaction, these products have not been demonstrated to improve analgesic outcomes.[29] In addition to sustained-release preparations, immediate-release medications should be continued to control breakthrough or incident pain at a dose typically 10% of the total 24-hour sustained-release dosage.

Opioid pharmacokinetics and pharmacodynamics

Numerous factors can affect the pharmacokinetics and pharmacodynamics of opioids, including factors associated with normal aging, such as a natural decline in organ function, and comorbidities, which are more common in elderly persons. A review of these issues follows.

Impact of normal aging Numerous well-documented pharmacokinetic alterations have been described as a result of the natural decline in the functioning of all organs caused by the normal aging process.[30] Reduced intravascular volume, organ volume, and muscle mass may alter drug distribution, resulting in increased plasma levels relative to that of a younger person.

The volume of distribution of fat-soluble opioids, namely fentanyl, may increase because of the increased fat-to-lean body mass ratio that accompanies aging, increasing the drug's effective half-life. The decreased volume of distribution that occurs owing to decreased total body water with aging may also result in increased plasma levels of more hydrophilic opioids (eg, morphine) compared with levels observed in younger persons.[30] In general, oral bioavailability does not seem to be affected by age, and although first-pass metabolism may be affected, dosage adjustments are not routinely necessary beyond the 25% to 50% dose reduction recommended at opioid initiation.[31]

Renal clearance (glomerular filtration, tubular reabsorption, and secretion) decreases with age by about 6% to 10% per decade beginning at age 30 years, so that by age 70 a person may have a 40% to 50% reduction in renal function without underlying kidney disease.[31,32] Opioid clearance may be significantly delayed because most opioids are highly reliant on renal elimination, with methadone and buprenorphine being noteworthy exceptions. Hepatic clearance is also reduced, affected mainly by the reduction of hepatic blood flow while hepatic enzyme activity is minimally impacted with age. Although the effects of aging itself may not dramatically impact the pharmacokinetics of opioids, increased sensitivity to opioid analgesics (or pharmacodynamic alterations) are observed in older adults, suggesting an altered intrinsic potency. Taken together, opioid use requires lower dosages and less frequent administration in the elderly.

Impact of comorbidities In addition to the altered intrinsic potency of opioids that are dependent on age, underlying comorbidities must also be considered before initiation of these agents.

Liver dysfunction Hepatitis, cirrhosis, or hepatic malignancies that significantly affect hepatic function can substantially increase opioid bioavailability, so close monitoring of dose effectiveness and duration of action is essential in these patients. In general, older adults with significant liver dysfunction should have initial opioid doses decreased by 50%, and the dosing interval should be doubled.[33]

Cardiovascular disease and renal function In addition to the normal decrease in renal clearance that occurs with age, comorbidities that increase in frequency with age, such as hypertension, diabetes, and vascular disease, can adversely affect renal function. Decrements in renal function may decrease the excretion of some neurotoxic opioid-related metabolites. This caution is particularly true for codeine, morphine, hydromorphone, and oxycodone, and dose adjustments with even low doses of these agents should be made accordingly, along with close monitoring for toxicity (eg, myoclonus).[34–36] In general, hydromorphone and oxycodone are preferred over codeine and morphine for use in patients with renal insufficiency.[36]

Codeine should be not be used in patients with a creatinine clearance of less than 30 mL/min/1.73 m^2 because there have been reports of substantial toxicity, even with relatively low doses. Oxycodone has several active metabolites that may accumulate in renal dysfunction, but is considered to be safer than morphine. Limited case reports and pharmacokinetic data suggest that fentanyl can be used at usual doses in mild to moderate renal insufficiency and in patients undergoing dialysis if the drug's use is accompanied by proper monitoring of respiratory and cardiovascular status, blood pressure, and heart rate.[36]

Methadone is primarily excreted in the feces; thus, it is considered safe for use in persons with renal insufficiency. However, equianalgesic ratios between morphine and methadone are dose dependent, the half-life is highly variable, and numerous drug interactions must be considered; therefore, methadone should be used only by practitioners experienced with this agent.[37] Buprenorphine is also excreted primarily in the feces and is considered safe in persons with renal impairment.[38]

Assessment and management of opioid-related risks and side effects One common reason cited for noncompliance with opioid therapy is the fear of side effects. The side effects of most concern include constipation, nausea and vomiting, sedation, confusion, and respiratory depression. Tolerance develops to most of these side effects, with the exception of constipation. Falls represent a more recent concern based on the findings of recent studies.[17] Given the heterogeneity of opioid-related side effects, older adults should be instructed not to drive until a steady state has been achieved and no impact on driving capabilities has developed. Reassurance to the patient coupled with proactive management of common side effects are key strategies for reducing complications and increasing adherence to opioid therapy.

Nausea develops in about one-third of patients initiated on opioids and occurs because these agents slow down the motility of the GI tract, stimulate the chemoreceptor trigger zone, and sensitize the vestibular apparatus. If severe nausea occurs, low-dose haloperidol (0.5 mg) or ondansetron (4 mg) scheduled or "as needed" typically manage nausea until it resolves over the first week of therapy. Opioid-related constipation should also be considered and treated if present when a patient on opioids presents with nausea.

Constipation is common in older persons with serious illnesses and nearly universal in patients taking an opioid, which is often cited by older adults as a reason to refuse opioid therapy. Constipation results from μ-receptor binding in the GI tract, resulting in slower transit time and subsequent increased water reabsorption. Prevention is the cornerstone of constipation management with a bowel stimulant of senna or bisacodyl scheduled daily at initiation and increased to twice daily if needed.[39] Osmotic agents, such as polyethylene glycol or milk of magnesia, as monotherapy generally lack sufficient action to counteract opioid GI effects, but can be helpful in conjunction with stimulant laxatives when needed. Bulk-forming agents such as psyllium are ineffective and can worsen symptoms if patients do not ingest an adequate amount of fluid.

The relationship between pain, falls, and opioids is complex and not completely understood. Cohort studies support that pain interference is associated with an increased risk of falls among community-dwelling older adults. At the same time, the use of opioids, particularly short acting, at time of initiation, may increase the likelihood of falls compared with those with arthritis pain treated with an NSAID.[40] However, published studies examining the relationship between analgesic use and falls have noteworthy limitations, including opioid patients reporting greater comorbidity versus comparison groups, as well as a lack of adjustment for starting opioid dose. The relationship among pain, cognition, and opioids also remains inconclusive. Undertreated pain may predispose to an increased likelihood of confusion, particularly in the hospital. For example, a study of hospitalized hip fracture patients found that persons taking higher opioid doses had a lower delirium risk compared with patients taking low-dose or no opioid.[41]

Black box warning

All opioids contain a black box warning for the risk of abuse, diversion, and fatal overdose owing to respiratory depression. Respiratory depression is rare in opioid-naive patients whose treatment is initiated at low doses. Risk has been shown to increase with age, opioid dose, and with underlying pulmonary conditions, such as chronic obstructive pulmonary disease and sleep apnea. The concomitant administration of opioids with other central nervous system depressants (eg, benzodiazepines, alcohol, barbiturates) can also significantly increase the risk of respiratory depression for which patients should be educated.

Any patient being considered for opioid therapy must be treated with "universal precautions" against addiction and misuse. Prescribers need to understand state laws and regulations when prescribing opioid therapy, because active legislation is ongoing in many states. Addiction and misuse is another cited reason why older adults may decline a trial of opioid therapy for the management of moderate to severe pain. Each patient requires risk stratification for addiction and misuse with adherence monitoring commensurate with risk. Patients at moderate or greater risk for addiction or misuse should be considered for referral to a pain specialist. Patients must be educated about safe drug storage and sharing, which is a federal crime.

To date, research on opioid addiction and the older adult is lacking, including prevalence data and risk factors. Available research suggests addiction risk is much lower in older adults compared with younger adults, but data specific to newer aging cohorts, such as the baby boomers, is lacking. Experts recommend asking about and documenting risk factors of addiction in younger persons, which include (1) personal or family history of alcohol and/or drug abuse, (2) a history of preadolescent sexual abuse, and (3) psychiatric disease. Opioid risk stratification tools may also be employed and are often recommended by guidelines to help identify and mitigate risk of addiction and misuse; however, research documenting their benefits and harms in primary care and older populations is lacking. Commonly used risk tools include the Screening Tool for Addiction Risk (STAR) and Screener and Opioid Assessment for Patients with Pain (SOAPP).

Adherence monitoring should be integrated into the pain management plan with patient risk of addiction and misuse determining which steps to incorporate into the care plan. For lower risk patients, adherence protocols may include monthly physician visits with pill counts, required use of only 1 pharmacy, home health to better supervise patients in the home setting, and documentation of pain-related outcomes. For higher risk patients, strategies may include urine toxicology screens; use of long-acting medications without breakthrough; prescribing small quantities at a time, although this strategy can be problematic with some insurance carriers (particularly Medicaid); prescribing opioids less prone to abuse such as methadone and buprenorphine; and use of a patient–prescriber agreement. Patient–prescriber agreements should not be thought of as punitive, but as an opportunity to openly discuss the benefits and risks of opioid therapy and how the provider and patient are going to work together to mitigate the risks.[42]

Nonopioid Analgesics

Duloxetine

Duloxetine is a serotonin and norepinephrine reuptake inhibitor with analgesic efficacy purportedly related to its central effect with influence on descending inhibition. Randomized, controlled studies have established the analgesic efficacy of duloxetine in 4 chronic pain conditions: diabetic peripheral neuropathy, fibromyalgia, chronic low back pain, and osteoarthritis knee pain.[43–45] Each of these studies predominately enrolled younger patients, with the exception of the knee pain studies, where the average patient age was in the mid 60s. FDA indications for use of duloxetine include each of these conditions, with the exception of chronic low back pain. Duloxetine is usually started at 30 mg/d and may be increased to 60 mg/d after 2 weeks if appropriate.

The most commonly experienced adverse events associated with duloxetine are dry mouth, nausea, constipation, diarrhea, fatigue, dizziness, somnolence, and insomnia. Nausea is typically mild to moderate in severity and generally resolves within 1 week. A small, statistically significant but clinically insignificant increase in hemoglobin A1C levels has been reported in the diabetic peripheral neuropathy studies with duloxetine use compared with placebo. Duloxetine should not be prescribed to patients with hepatic impairment or heavy alcohol use because cases of elevated liver enzymes, hepatitis, jaundice, and hepatic failure have been reported.

Given the available evidence, duloxetine may be considered for the management of moderate to severe, persistent pain from osteoarthritis of the knees or back where acetaminophen or opioids have been unsuccessful (duloxetine monotherapy) or not provided enough relief (combination therapy with addition of duloxetine).

Gabapentin and pregabalin

Gabapentin and pregabalin are antiepileptic drugs that, through alterations in ascending nociceptive pathways, have been shown to be effective in the management of several painful neuropathic conditions that occur commonly in older adults.

Gabapentin carries FDA indications for post-herpetic neuralgia, whereas pregabalin has FDA indications for post-herpetic neuralgia, diabetic peripheral neuropathy, fibromyalgia, and neuropathic pain associated with spinal cord injury. Both of these medications have few drug interactions.[46] They are excreted renally as unchanged drug and dose reduction with renal insufficiency is necessary. Gabapentin dosing requires slow titration starting at doses as low as 100 mg/d. The dose can be increased every 3 to 7 days based on analgesic response and tolerance up to maximum dosage of 3600 mg/d in divided doses. This process can take several months. Pregabalin can be titrated more easily. The starting dose is 100 mg/d and increased incrementally to 300 mg/d over several weeks if necessary. The medication is given in 2 or 3 divided doses. Dizziness, sedation, and peripheral edema are the most common side effects and are more common in older adults.

Gabapentin and pregabalin therapy should be considered first line agents or for use as co-analgesics among older adults with post-herpetic neuralgia and/or diabetic peripheral neuropathy. Clinicians should start at a low dose and increase slowly the dose every few days until desired analgesia is achieved, limiting side effects emerge, or the maximum recommended dose is reached. As with opioids, older adults should abstain from driving until a steady state has been achieved and no impact on driving capabilities has developed.

Topical Therapies

Topical nonsteroidal anti-inflammatory drugs

Even though oral NSAIDs are effective for the management of mild pain, significant adverse GI, cardiovascular, and renal effects, particularly in the older population limit their widespread use. Topical NSAIDs represent an alternative to oral NSAIDs, so that patients may benefit from local analgesia with lower risk of systemic adverse effects.[47] In the United States, 2 topical diclofenac formulations, namely, diclofenac sodium 1% topical gel and diclofenac sodium 1.5% topical solution, have been approved for the treatment of osteoarthritis pain. Diclofenac epolamine 1.3% topical patch has also been approved for the treatment of pain owing to minor strains and sprains. A recent Cochrane review reported topical NSAIDs were as effective as oral NSAIDs for the relief of chronic musculoskeletal pain with fewer systemic adverse effects, particularly in hand and knee osteoarthritis.[48]

Capsaicin

Capsaicin, primarily studied for the management of neuropathic pain, is derived from the chili pepper and stimulates the ion of the transient receptor potential vanilloid-1 (TRPV1). It is available as a topical agent in a low dose (0.075%) applied several times a day for several weeks and a high-dose (8%), 1-time preparation that may be repeated. Upon application to the skin, a brief initial sensitization is followed by prolonged desensitization with depletion of substance P. Although low-dose capsaicin has not resulted in good efficacy, the larger dose 8% topical capsaicin has had some benefit in select patients for the treatment of post-herpetic neuralgia and HIV neuropathic pain.[49,50]

Topical lidocaine

Lidocaine 5% topical patch has been shown to be safe, effective, and well-tolerated for the treatment for post-herpetic neuralgia. Although it may be reasonable to use a topical lidocaine patch for similarly focal neuropathic pains, such as post-thoracotomy pain, we strongly recommend against its use for other painful conditions, including osteoarthritis and back pain, given a lack of evidence demonstrating efficacy.[51] Placement is advised for only 12 hours daily; however, pharmacokinetic studies of use up to

24 hours demonstrate minimal systemic absorption. The most common side effects are mild skin reactions and no drug–drug interactions have been reported in clinical trials.[51]

SUMMARY

Persistent pain in older adults is a common problem linked to significant morbidity. Effective pain management begins with thorough and multidimensional assessment and goal setting. Normal physiologic changes and the impact of comorbidity have to be considered in both the selection of analgesic agents and their initial and subsequent dosing. Successful medication management is possible with attention to detail, careful titration, and monitoring of analgesic effect and adverse effects.

REFERENCES

1. Shega JW, Tiedt A, Grant K, et al. Pain measurement in the national social life, health, and aging project (NSHAP): presence, intensity, and location. J Gerontol B Psychol Sci Soc Sci 2014;69(Suppl 2):S191–7.
2. Maxwell CJ, Dalby DM, Slater M, et al. The prevalence and management of current daily pain among older home care clients. Pain 2008;138(1):208–16.
3. Smith AK, Cenzer IS, Knight SJ, et al. The epidemiology of pain during the last 2 years of life. Ann Intern Med 2010;153(9):563–9.
4. AGS Panel on Persistent Pain in Older Persons. The management of persistent pain in older persons. J Am Geriatr Soc 2002;50(Suppl 6):S205–24.
5. Weiner DK, Haggerty CL, Kritchvesky SB, et al. How does low back pain impact physical function in independent, well-functioning older adults? Evidence from the Health ABC Cohort and implications for the future. Pain Med 2003;4(4): 311–20.
6. Bosley BN, Weiner DK, Rudy TE, et al. Is chronic nonmalignant pain associated with decreased appetite in older adults? Preliminary evidence. J Am Geriatr Soc 2004;52:247–51.
7. Shega JW, Dale W, Andrews M, et al. Persistent pain and frailty: a case for pain homeostenosis? J Am Geriatr Soc 2012;60(1):113–7.
8. Shega JW, Andrew M, Lau D, et al. The relationship between persistent pain and 5-year mortality: a population-based, prospective cohort study. J Am Geriatr Soc 2013;61(12):2135–40.
9. Sawyer P, Bodner EV, Ritchie CS, et al. Pain and pain medication use in community-dwelling older adults. Am J Geriatr Pharmacother 2006;4(4):316–24.
10. Won AB, Lapane KL, Vallow S, et al. Persistent nonmalignant pain and analgesic prescribing patterns in elderly nursing home residents. J Am Geriatr Soc 2004; 52(6):867–74.
11. Bernabei R, Gambassi G, Lapane K, et al. Management of pain in elderly patients with cancer. SAGE Study Group. Systematic Assessment of Geriatric Drug Use via Epidemiology. JAMA 1998;279(23):1877–82 [Erratum appears in JAMA 1999;281(2):136].
12. Herr K. Pain assessment strategies in older adults. J Pain 2011;12(3):s3–13.
13. Herr K, Coyne PJ, Key T, et al. Pain assessment in the nonverbal patient: position statement with clinical practice recommendations. Pain Manag Nurs 2006;7(2): 44–52.
14. Trescot AM, Helm S, Hansen H, et al. Opioids in the management of chronic non-cancer pain: an update of American Society of the Interventional Pain Physicians' (ASIPP) Guidelines. Pain Physician 2008;11(Suppl 2):S5–62.

15. Papaleontiou M, Henderson CR Jr, Turner BJ, et al. Outcomes associated with opioid use in the treatment of chronic noncancer pain in older adults: a systematic review and meta-analysis. J Am Geriatr Soc 2010;58(7):1353–69.
16. Gilron I, Bailey JM, Tu D, et al. Morphine, gabapentin, or their combination for neuropathic pain. N Engl J Med 2005;352:1324–34.
17. Rolita L, Spegman A, Tang X, et al. Greater number of narcotic analgesic prescriptions for osteoarthritis is associated with falls and fractures in elderly adults. J Am Geriatr Soc 2013;61(3):335–40.
18. Jahr JS, Breitmeyer JB, Pan C, et al. Safety and efficacy of Intravenous acetaminophen in the elderly after major orthopedic surgery: subset data analysis from 3, randomized, placebo-controlled trials. Am J Ther 2012;19(2):66–75.
19. Graham GG, Davies MJ, Day RO, et al. The modern pharmacology of paracetamol: therapeutic actions, mechanism of action, metabolism, toxicity and recent pharmacological findings. Inflammopharmacology 2013;21:201–32.
20. Larson AM, Polson J, Fontana RJ, et al. Acute Liver Failure Study Group. Acetaminophen-induced acute liver failure: results of a US multicenter prospective study. Hepatology 2005;42(6):1364–72.
21. U.S Food and Drug Administration. FDA Drug Safety Communication: Prescription acetaminophen products to be limited to 325 mg per dosage unit; boxed warning will highlight potential for severe liver failure. January 13, 2011. Available at: http://www.fda.gov/Drugs/DrugSafety/ucm239821.htm. Accessed December 11, 2014.
22. American Geriatrics Society Panel on the Pharmacological Management of Persistent Pain in Older Persons. Pharmacological management of persistent pain in older persons. J Am Geriatr Soc 2009;57(8):1331–46.
23. Barkin RL, Beckerman M, Blum SL, et al. Should nonsteroidal anti-inflammatory drugs (NSAIDs) be prescribed to the older adult? Drugs Aging 2010;27(10):775–89.
24. Wallace MB, Durlaski VL, Vaughn J, et al. Age and alarm symptoms do not predict endoscopic findings among patients with dyspepsia: a multicenter database study. Gut 2001;49:29–34.
25. Pilotto A, Franceschi M, Leandro G, et al. Proton pump inhibitors reduce the risk of uncomplicated peptic ulcer in the elderly either acute or chronic users of aspirin/nonsteroidal anti-inflammatory drugs. Aliment Pharmacol Ther 2004;20:1091–7.
26. Pilotto A, Franceschi M, Leandro G, et al. The risk of upper gastrointestinal bleeding in the elderly users of aspirin and other nonsteroidal anti-inflammatory drugs: the role of gastroprotective drugs. Aging Clin Exp Res 2003;15:494–9.
27. Reddy A, Yennurajalingam S, Pulivarthi K, et al. Frequency, outcome, and predictors of success within 6 weeks of an opioid rotation among outpatients with cancer receiving strong opioids. Oncologist 2013;18:212–20.
28. Gupta DK, Avram MJ. Rational opioid dosing in the elderly: dose and dosing intervals when initiating opioid therapy. Clin Pharmacol Ther 2012;91(2):339–43.
29. Rauck RL. What is the case for prescribing long-acting over short-acting opioids for patients with chronic pain? A critical review. Pain Pract 2009;9(6):468–79.
30. Schwartz JB. The current state of knowledge on age, sex, and their interactions on clinical pharmacology. Clin Pharmacol Ther 2007;82(1):87–96.
31. Tumer N, Scarpace PJ, Lowenthal DT. Geriatric pharmacology: basic and clinical considerations. Annu Rev Pharmacol Toxicol 1992;32:271–302.
32. Davies DF, Shock NW. Age changes in glomerular filtration rate, effect of venal plasma flow, and tubular excretory capacity in adult males. J Clin Invest 1950;29(5):496–507.

33. Verbeeck RK. Pharmacokinetics and dose adjustments in patients with hepatic dysfunction. Eur J Clin Pharmacol 2008;64(12):1147–61.
34. Murtagh FE, Chai MO, Donohoe P, et al. The use of opioid analgesia in end-stage renal disease patients managed without dialysis: recommendations for practice. J Pain Palliat Care Pharmacother 2007;21(2):5–16.
35. Pham PC, Toscano E, Pham PM, et al. Pain management in patients with chronic kidney disease. NDT Plus 2009;2(2):111–8.
36. Dean M. Opioids in renal failure and dialysis patients. J Pain Symptom Manage 2004;28(5):497–504.
37. Lugo RA, Satterfield KL, Kern SE. Pharmacokinetics of methadone. J Pain Palliat Care Pharmacother 2005;19(4):13–24.
38. Vadivelu N, Hines RL. Management of chronic pain in the elderly: focus on transdermal buprenorphine. Clin Interv Aging 1998;3(3):421–30.
39. Cherny N, Ripamonti C, Pereira J, et al. Strategies to manage the adverse effects of oral morphine: an evidence-based report. J Clin Oncol 2001;19(9):2542–54.
40. Miller M, Stürmer T, Azrael D, et al. Opioid analgesics and the risk of fractures among older adults with arthritis. J Am Geriatr Soc 2011;59(3):430–8.
41. Morrison RS, Magaziner J, Gilbert M, et al. Relationship between pain and opioid analgesics on the development of delirium following hip fracture. J Gerontol A Biol Sci Med Sci 2003;58A(1):76–81.
42. Chou R, Fanciullo GJ, Fine PG, et al. Opioid treatment guidelines: clinical guidelines for the use of chronic opioid therapy in chronic non-cancer pain. J Pain 2009;10(2):113–30.
43. Brown JP, Boulay LJ. Clinical experience with duloxetine in the management of chronic musculoskeletal pain. A focus on osteoarthritis of the knee. Ther Adv Musculoskelet Dis 2013;5(6):291–304.
44. Smith T, Nicholson RA. Review of duloxetine in the management of diabetic peripheral neuropathic pain. Vasc Health Risk Manag 2007;3(6):833–44.
45. Wright CL, Mist CD, Ross RL, et al. Duloxetine for the treatment of fibromyalgia. Expert Rev Clin Immunol 2010;6(5):745–56.
46. Haslam C, Nurmikko T. Pharmacological treatment of neuropathic pain in older persons. Clin Interv Aging 2008;3(1):111–20.
47. Balmaceda CM. Clinical trial data in support of changing guidelines in osteoarthritis treatment. J Pain Res 2014;7:211–8.
48. Derry S, Moore RA, Rabbie R. Topical NSAIDs for chronic musculoskeletal pain in adults. Cochrane Database Syst Rev 2012;(9):CD007400.
49. Derry S, Sven-Rice A, Cole P, et al. Topical capsaicin (high concentration) for chronic neuropathic pain in adults. Cochrane Database Syst Rev 2013;(2):CD007393.
50. Derry S, Moore RA. Topical capsaicin (low concentration) for chronic neuropathic pain in adults. Cochrane Database Syst Rev 2012;(9):CD010111.
51. Derry S, Wiffen PJ, Moore RA, et al. Topical lidocaine for neuropathic pain in adults [review]. Cochrane Database Syst Rev 2014;(7):CD010958.
52. Smith H. Opioid metabolism. Mayo Clin Proc 2009;84(7):613–24.
53. Trescot AM, Datta S, Lee M, et al. Opioid pharmacology. Pain Physician 2008; 11(Suppl 2):S133–53.
54. Pergolizzi J, Boger RH, Budd K, et al. Opioids and the management of chronic severe pain in the elderly: consensus statement of an International Expert Panel with focus on the six clinically most often used World Health Organization Step III opioids (buprenorphine, fentanyl, hydromorphone, methadone, morphine, and oxycodone. Pain Pract 2008;8(4):287–313.

Management of Diabetes in the Elderly

Nidhi Bansal, MBBS, Ruban Dhaliwal, MD, Ruth S. Weinstock, MD, PhD*

KEYWORDS

- Diabetes mellitus • Geriatric • Insulin • Hypoglycemia • Frailty • Hypertension

KEY POINTS

- Glycemic and blood pressure goals need to be individualized and focused on avoidance of symptomatic hyperglycemia, hypoglycemia, orthostatic hypotension, and other adverse drug effects.
- Presence of geriatric syndromes, major comorbidities, frailty, advanced age, and social support must be considered in the management plan.
- Initial therapy for type 2 diabetes, in the absence of renal insufficiency, is low-dose metformin. The more expensive dipeptidyl peptidase 4 inhibitors are also well tolerated.
- If a sulfonylurea is to be used, consider short-acting glipizide. Insulin, when needed, should be used cautiously, because serious hypoglycemia can be a major problem in the elderly.
- Patient safety, preference, and preservation of quality of life should be primary objectives.

INTRODUCTION

An increasing number of older adults are newly diagnosed with diabetes, and an increasing population have diabetes of greater than 20 years duration. Although type 2 diabetes is most common in the geriatric age group, there are also more older adults than ever with long-standing type 1 diabetes. They have unique and diverse needs and challenges, which should be considered when developing a treatment plan. The approach to management of diabetes in the elderly must be individualized and changed over time depending on the presence and progression of geriatric syndromes, comorbidities, and risk of hypoglycemia. Availability of social support and personal preferences are also important. Current guidelines for the management of diabetes in the geriatric population are reviewed in this article.

Disclosure: R.S. Weinstock: Participation in multicenter clinical trials sponsored by Medtronic, Sanofi, Novo Nordisk, Intarcia and Eli Lilly.
Department of Medicine, Division of Endocrinology, Diabetes and Metabolism, SUNY Upstate Medical University, 750 East Adams Street, Syracuse, NY 13210, USA
* Corresponding author.
E-mail address: weinstor@upstate.edu

Med Clin N Am 99 (2015) 351–377
http://dx.doi.org/10.1016/j.mcna.2014.11.008
0025-7125/15/$ – see front matter © 2015 Elsevier Inc. All rights reserved.

DIABETES IN OLDER ADULTS: OVERVIEW
Incidence and Prevalence of Diabetes and Associated Chronic Complications

Increasing incidence and improving life expectancy have led to an increase in prevalence of diabetes in the geriatric age group.[1,2] In the United States in 2012, 29.1 million people, 9.3% of the total population, had diabetes, generating $245 billion in diabetes-related costs.[1] Of those 65 years of age or older, an estimated 11.2 million (25.9%) had diabetes. The rate of new diagnoses per 1000 was 11.5%, representing 400,000 new cases in 2012.[1] The prevalence of diabetes in skilled nursing facilities is even higher.[3]

The development of the microvascular complications of diabetes (retinopathy, neuropathy, and nephropathy) are related, in large part, to glycemic control and disease duration. Although better glycemic control and earlier detection and treatment of retinopathy and macular edema have helped reduce visual loss and blindness from diabetes, vision impairment remains a larger problem in adults 60 years of age or older with diabetes compared with those without diabetes.[4]

The presence of peripheral neuropathy contributes to difficulties with ambulation and greater propensity for falls. Neuropathies as well as peripheral vascular disease are also risk factors for amputations. Diabetes-related amputations declined between 1990 and 2010.[5] This decrease is probably related to many factors, including better foot care (improved prevention, early detection and treatment of foot infections and ulcers), reduction in smoking, and improved glycemic control. In 2010, the incidence of amputations (per 10,000) was 37.3 and 36.0 in those aged 65 to 74 years and 75 years and older.[5] These rates are 5.9 and 2.7 times higher than for adults aged 65 to 74 years and 75 years and older without diabetes.

The incidence of end-stage renal disease (ESRD) in people with diabetes increased from 1990 to 2010.[5] In 2010, the incidence (per 10,000) was 30.5 and 28.6 in those aged 65 to 74 years and 75 years and older, respectively, representing a 3.7 and 2.1 higher incidence compared with those without diabetes in these age groups. Older adults in 2010 also had more ESRD compared with younger people with diabetes, with a greater events difference (per 10,000) in those aged 75 years and older compared with those aged 65 to 74 years (12.3 and 2.9, respectively). This situation is despite better treatment to prevent or forestall ESRD with use of angiotensin-converting enzyme inhibitors (ACE-I) or angiotensin receptor blockers (ARBs), and better blood pressure and blood glucose control. There are undoubtedly multiple contributing factors. These incidence rates for ESRD are based on initiation of ESRD treatment. It is possible that the higher reported incidence of ESRD in the geriatric population is related, in part, to more elderly people receiving treatment of ESRD.

The macrovascular complications of diabetes (cardiovascular, cerebrovascular, and peripheral arterial disease) are major causes of morbidity and mortality and contribute to the rate of physical disability observed in many older adults with diabetes, although there is some evidence that rates of these complications may be decreasing in the elderly.[4] Acute myocardial infarctions and strokes (events difference per 10,000) decreased significantly from 1990 to 2010, with the relative differences being even greater in those aged 75 years and older than in those aged 65 to 74 years.[5] The magnitude of the reduction was greatest for acute myocardial infarctions and stroke, possibly related to better clinical care and identification and treatment of risk factors (eg, use of statins and blood pressure medications and smoking cessation).

Glycemic Control in Older Adults

Glycemic control in people 65 years of age and older has improved in the past 2 decades. Comparing results from the National Health and Nutrition Examination Surveys of 1988 to 1994 and 1999 to 2010, the percentage of adults aged 65 years and older with A_{1c} levels less than 7.0% and less than 8.0% is higher. This finding was associated with greater use of both oral glycemic control medications and insulin.[2] In 2005 to 2010, for adults aged 65 years and older with diabetes, of those with A_{1c} levels less than 7.0% (65.9%) and less than 8.0% (88.7%), diabetes medications were being taken by 62.5% and 87.4%, respectively: insulin alone 12.9%, oral agents alone 60.5%, insulin + oral agents 15.4%, and no medications 11.2%.[2] It is unknown how many of those taking insulin alone had type 1 diabetes.

Studies in older patients with diabetes suggest increased risk of morbidity and mortality at both low and high A_{1c} levels.[6,7] Results from the Diabetes and Aging Study suggest higher mortality with A_{1c} levels less than 6.0% and greater than 9.0%, and increased diabetes complications with A_{1c} levels 8.0% or higher.[7] In the ACCORD (Action to Control Cardiovascular Risk in Diabetes) study, the older participants had more hypoglycemia.[8] It is becoming increasingly clear that overtreatment, particularly in older adults, is a significant problem.[9]

Severe Hypoglycemia in Older Adults

As older adults with diabetes achieve better metabolic control, in part through the use of medications that can cause hypoglycemia, hospitalizations and death caused by hyperglycemia have declined, but serious hypoglycemia is a growing concern.[2,5,10] Medicare beneficiaries 75 years of age and older were twice as likely to experience a hospitalization between 1999 and 2011 as a result of hypoglycemia as those aged 65 to 74 years.[10] When examining emergency department visits and hospitalizations from 2007 to 2011, those 80 years of age and older had the highest number of emergency department visits for insulin-related hypoglycemia (34.9/1000 insulin-treated patients); compared with 45-year-olds to 64-year-olds with diabetes, they were almost 5 times more likely to require hospitalization.[11] Insulin errors causing these events included taking too much short-acting insulin for the mealtime food intake, taking the wrong insulin dose, using the wrong insulin product (mixing up the long-acting and short-acting insulins), taking insulin at the wrong time of day, and taking too much insulin to correct for hyperglycemia. Older adults hospitalized with hypoglycemia have higher morbidity and mortality than younger adults.[12]

Most research on older adults with diabetes has focused on type 2 diabetes. Studies examining insulin-requiring diabetes and hypoglycemia in the geriatric population frequently do not distinguish between type 2 diabetes (most of the geriatric diabetes population) and type 1 diabetes. However, the prevalence of type 1 diabetes in older adults is also increasing. Information from the Type 1 Diabetes Exchange registry indicates that 21% of adults aged 65 years and older with duration of type 1 diabetes of at least 40 years self-report having had a seizure or loss of consciousness from hypoglycemia over the previous 12 months.[13] Severe hypoglycemia was more likely with A_{1c} levels less than 7.0% and with A_{1c} levels greater than 7.5%. Severe hypoglycemia was as common in poorly controlled (A_{1c} levels 8%–9%) as it was in well-controlled (A_{1c} level <6.5%) type 1 diabetes.

Risk Factors, Symptoms, and Consequences of Hypoglycemia

Insulin therapy is the major risk factor for serious hypoglycemia. Insulin dosing errors occur in the presence of poor cognition, erratic eating, and impairment of vision and dexterity. Treatment with insulin secretagogues, especially long-acting sulfonylurea drugs, is also associated with severe hypoglycemia in the geriatric population. Deterioration in renal function usually requires adjustment in dosing, because most of the drugs have renal clearance. Poor nutritional status and renal or hepatic impairment can result in impaired mobilization of glucose (in part because of lower glycogen stores and impaired gluconeogenesis) during hypoglycemia. In addition, loss of adrenergic responses to hypoglycemia in the elderly can contribute to more serious hypoglycemic episodes. The most important risk factors for hypoglycemia are shown in **Table 1**.

Because older adults may have impaired counterregulatory responses to hypoglycemia, they can lack the usual autonomic warning signs of hypoglycemia (eg, tremulousness, palpitations, sweating). It is important to recognize and avoid hypoglycemia. Symptoms that can indicate hypoglycemia as well as potential serious consequences are listed in **Table 1**. Because the symptoms of hypoglycemia are frequently nonspecific, blood glucose levels should be tested to confirm hypoglycemia.

MANAGEMENT GOALS
Geriatric-Specific Considerations

The presence of geriatric syndromes, including frailty, cognitive impairment, poor mobility, dexterity, and balance, reduced vision and hearing, depression, and chronic pain, need to be assessed, as described in the article by Carlson and colleagues elsewhere in this issue. Older adults also need to be evaluated for urinary incontinence, polypharmacy, nutritional status, falls, numeracy and literacy skills, treatment adherence, social support, and home safety. These conditions, as well as the presence of other comorbid conditions, such as cardiovascular disease (CVD), cerebrovascular disease, chronic kidney disease, and neuropathy, must be considered when formulating therapeutic approaches and treatment goals.[27]

Table 1		
Hypoglycemia in older adults with diabetes		
Risk Factors	**Symptoms**	**Consequences**
• Older age (>80 y)	Neuroglycopenic	• Impaired cognition
• Type 1 diabetes of >20 y duration	Confusion and/or disorientation	• Coma
• Insulin treatment	Unsteady gait and/or falls	• Seizures
• Use of insulin secretagogues, especially sulfonylurea drugs	Difficulty speaking and/or concentrating	• Cardiac arrhythmias and other cardiac events
• History of severe hypoglycemia	Impaired vision, blurred or double vision	• Hospitalizations
• Hypoglycemic unawareness or poor hypoglycemic awareness	Fatigue and/or drowsiness	• Accidents
• Reduced renal function	Lightheadedness	• Depression
• Hepatic insufficiency	Feeling weak and/or dizzy	• Difficulty with ambulation
• Alcohol use	Loss of consciousness	• Difficulty reading
• Poor nutritional status	Autonomic	• Unsteady gait
• Unpredictable food intake	Tremulousness	• Falls and fractures
• Polypharmacy	Hunger and/or nausea	• Increased risk of dementia
• Frailty/poor visual-motor skills	Anxiety and/or feeling tearful	• Reduced quality of life
• Cognitive dysfunction or dementia	Palpitations	
• Depression	Feeling warm or sweaty	

Data from Refs.[13–26]

Glycemic Goals

Because there are few studies comparing diabetes management approaches in older adults, most recommendations are based on expert opinion. Guidelines for glycemic treatment focus on A_{1c} goals, but even in the presence of a high A_{1c} level, the individual may be having serious hypoglycemic episodes.[13] Review of blood glucose levels is important to detect wide glycemic excursions. Especially with insulin therapy, home glucose monitoring is essential and should help direct therapy. A_{1c} levels may also be misleading in the presence of anemia, renal disease, recent blood loss, and any other condition associated with shortened red blood cell life span.

Goals recommended by different professional groups and associations are summarized in **Table 2**. There is agreement that goals should be individualized, taking into account the overall health status, presence of comorbid conditions and frailty, cognitive status, presence of hypoglycemic unawareness, history of hypoglycemia, life expectancy, available social support, and patient preference. Older adults in excellent health, without functional or cognitive limitations, who desire good glycemic control, can follow guidelines developed for younger adults. Glycemic goals for older adults who are frail, functionally dependent, and have serious comorbidities should be individualized, using higher A_{1c} goals that are acceptable to patients and caregivers, avoiding symptomatic hyperglycemia.

Blood Pressure Goals

Blood pressure goals may be higher in older adults based on their functional and cognitive status, comorbidities, polypharmacy, and life expectancy. Recommendations are shown in **Table 2**. In general, healthy older adults with diabetes and without major comorbidities should aim for blood pressure less than 140/80 mm Hg, whereas for the frail elderly with functional and cognitive impairment and limited life expectancy, the blood pressure goal should be less than 150/90 mm Hg. A systolic blood pressure less than 140 mm Hg may be appropriate in older adults with evidence of renal impairment (estimated glomerular filtration rate [eGFR] <60 mL/min/1.73 m^2).[31]

Low-Density Lipoprotein Cholesterol Goals

Goals in the treatment of hyperlipidemia are shown in **Table 2**. With the exception of those with limited life expectancy and individuals who cannot tolerate statin drugs, statin therapy is generally recommended. The American Diabetes Association recommendations state that all individuals older than 40 years with diabetes should be treated with a statin drug if they have at least 1 additional cardiovascular risk factor (hypertension, smoking, dyslipidemia, albuminuria, or family history of CVD),[38] but statin use in those older than 80 years remains controversial.[39] Low doses of statin drugs can be used to reduce side effects and drug-drug interactions.

PHARMACOLOGIC STRATEGIES

Most older adults with diabetes have type 2 diabetes, most of whom can be treated with oral agents. However, some require insulin therapy, as do all with type 1 diabetes. Type 2 diabetes in the elderly is heterogeneous; some individuals are lean and others obese, some are insulin sensitive and others resistant, and their degree of frailty can vary, necessitating individualized treatment plans. In general, pharmacologic therapy should be initiated with the lowest possible dose. In the presence of geriatric syndromes, additional behavioral interventions may be helpful to increase the overall success of the treatment plan (**Table 3**).

Table 2
Management goals in elderly with diabetes

Guidelines	Glycemic Goals	Blood Pressure Goal (mm Hg)	LDL Cholesterol Goal (mg/dL)	Recommendations for Statin Therapy
American Diabetes Association/American Geriatric Society	Healthy A_{1c} <7.5% Fasting/preprandial BG: 90–130 mg/dL Bedtime BG: 90–150 mg/dL	<140/80	<100 In the presence of CVD: <70	Statin therapy recommended unless contraindicated or not tolerated
	Frail with complex/intermediate health (several chronic illnesses or mild to moderate cognitive impairment or 2+ instrumental ADL deficits) A_{1c} <8.0% Fasting/preprandial BG: 90–150 mg/dL Bedtime BG: 100–180 mg/dL	<140/80		Statin therapy recommended unless contraindicated or not tolerated
	Frail with poor health (end-stage chronic disease or moderate to severe cognitive impairment or 2+ ADL deficits) A_{1c} <8.5% Fasting/preprandial BG: 100–180 mg/dL Bedtime BG: 110–200 mg/dL	<150/90		Statin therapy recommended unless limited life expectancy, contraindicated or not tolerated
	Long-term care facility residents A_{1c} <8.5% Fasting/preprandial BG: 100–180 mg/dL Bedtime BG: 110–200 mg/dL	<150/90		Consider benefit with limited life expectancy
European Society of Cardiology/European Association for the Study of Diabetes	A_{1c} <8.0%	<140/85 In presence of nephropathy: systolic BP <130	<100; In the presence of CVD, severe CKD or with 1 or more cardiovascular risk factors and/or target organ damage: <70 or at least ≥50% LDL reduction	Statin therapy recommended unless contraindicated or not tolerated

Organization	Glycemic target	BP target	LDL target	Statin
International Diabetes Federation	Functionally independent: $A_{1c} \leq 7.5\%$ Functionally dependent: $A_{1c} \leq 8.0\%$ Frail or dementia: $A_{1c} \leq 8.5\%$	<140/90 <150/90	<80 In the presence of CVD: <70 Frail or dementia: LDL goal can be relaxed	All older people with diabetes are at high CVD risk and should be considered for treatment with a statin unless contraindicated or considered clinically inappropriate Nonatherosclerotic dementia: appropriateness of statin use should be considered
International Association of Gerontology and Geriatrics/European Diabetes Working Party for Older People/International Task Force of Experts in Diabetes	Healthy: $A_{1c} \leq 7.5\%$ Frail (with major comorbidities: functionally dependent, multisystem disease, home care residency, with dementia): $A_{1c} \leq 8.5\%$	<140/80 Frail or those aged ≥75 y: <150/90	—	—

(continued on next page)

Table 2
(continued)

Guidelines		Glycemic Goals	Blood Pressure Goal (mm Hg)	LDL Cholesterol Goal (mg/dL)	Recommendations for Statin Therapy
Department of Veterans Affairs/Department of Defense	No major comorbidity or >10 y of life expectancy	Microvascular complications: Absent/mild: A_{1c} <7.0% Moderate: A_{1c} <8.0% Advanced: A_{1c} ≤9.0%	<140/80	<130 In the presence of CVD: <100	Statin therapy recommended if LDL level higher than goal, unless contraindicated or not tolerated LDL reduction of 30%–40% from baseline may be considered an alternative therapeutic strategy for patients who cannot meet the goals
	Major comorbidity present or 5–10 y of life expectancy	Microvascular complications: Absent, mild, or moderate: A_{1c} <8.0% Advanced: A_{1c} ≤9.0%			
	Marked (end-stage) comorbidity present or <5 y of life expectancy	A_{1c} ≤9.0%			

Abbreviations: A_{1c}, hemoglobin A_{1c}; ADL, activities of daily living; BG, blood glucose; BP, blood pressure; CKD, chronic kidney disease; LDL, low-density lipoprotein.
Data from Refs.[28-37]

Table 3
Diabetes self-management tasks in the elderly with geriatric syndromes

Self-Management Task	Geriatric Syndrome Affecting Self-Management	Possible Interventions
Self-monitoring of blood glucose	Vision and/or hearing impairment	Audio reminders (eg, devices with alarms)
		Use of talking home blood glucose monitoring devices
		Provide instructions printed in large font and with enhanced contrast
		Referral for vision and/or hearing aids
		Visual reminders (eg, erase board for refrigerator)
	Depression	Antidepressants
		Referral to mental health professional
	Diabetes-related distress	Simplification of regimen if possible
		Referral to diabetes educator/nurse
		Increased attention from educators (frequent visits or phone calls between office visits)
		Social services referral
Oral medication administration	Vision and/or hearing impairment and/or cognitive dysfunction	Audio reminders (eg, pill reminder dispensers/devices/organizers with alarms, including audio reminders)
		Simplify medication regimen
		Visual reminders (eg, erase board for refrigerator)
		Medication reminder applications on smart phones
		Medication reminder call services
	Low health literacy	Simplify medication regimen
		Provide instructions and education materials in appropriate format (eg, picture guides)
	Polypharmacy	Titrate medication dose (use lowest doses possible)
		Discontinue inappropriate medications and those no longer needed
		Review possible adverse effects of medications on glycemia, perception of hypoglycemia and geriatric syndromes
		Pharmacy assistance program
	Mobility issues	Mobility assistive devices (eg, cane, walker)
		Pharmacy delivery program
		Transportation assistance
		Social services
		Physical and occupational therapy consultations

(continued on next page)

Table 3
(continued)

Self-Management Task	Geriatric Syndrome Affecting Self-Management	Possible Interventions
	Diabetes-related distress	Simplification of regimen if possible
		Referral to diabetes educator/nurse
		Increased attention by educators (frequent visits or phone calls between office visits)
		Social services
Insulin administration and avoidance of serious hypoglycemia	Hypoglycemia unawareness or poor awareness	Diabetes self-management education
		Availability of rapidly absorbable carbohydrate; caretaker/partner instruction in use of glucagon (0.5–1 mg intramuscularly for severe hypoglycemia)
		Blood glucose awareness training
		Frequent blood glucose monitoring
		Use of personal continuous glucose monitoring systems
		Use of advanced insulin pump features (eg, low glucose threshold suspend)
		Adjustment of glucose targets
		Adjust timing of insulin administration
		Medical Alert bracelet or necklace and use of a medical alert system
	Vision and/or hearing impairment and/or cognitive dysfunction	Diabetes self-management education
		Audio reminders (eg, devices with alarms)
		Magnifier fitted for insulin syringes and/or insulin pump screen
		Hand or wallet magnifiers
		Use of insulin pens (count clicks for dosing)
		Improved lighting
		Provide instructions printed in large font and with enhanced contrast
		Use of dark-colored paper under the syringe/pen (to provide contrast)
		Visual reminders (eg, erase board for refrigerator)
		Simplification of medication regimen
		Use of a medical alert system
		Use of vibration and memory features on pumps
		Use of insulin pens with memory function
		Insulin vial stabilizers and needle guides

Low health literacy	Provide instructions and education materials in appropriate format (eg, picture guides)
Poor numeracy skills	Simplification of regimen
	Use of insulin dosing calculator
	Use of insulin pens
	Increase social support
Dexterity issues	Grip assistance products for syringes
	Injection aids
Chronic pain	Adequate pain management
Nutrition	Dietary counseling
	Simplify regimen (eg, change from carbohydrate counting to carbohydrate consistency)
	Social services (eg, need for Meals on Wheels, home care)
	Consider fixed mealtime insulin dosing (if eating is reliable and consistent meals can be provided)
	Consider rapidly acting insulin after the meal (reduce dose for poor food intake)
Depression	Antidepressants
	Referral to mental health professional
Mobility issues	Mobility assistive devices (eg, cane, walker)
	Pharmacy assistance program
	Pharmacy delivery program
	Transportation assistance
	Physical and occupational therapy consultations
	Social services
Diabetes-related distress	Simplification of regimen
	Referral to diabetes educator/nurse
	Increased attention by educators (frequent visits or phone calls between office visits)
Foot care Peripheral neuropathy	Proper footwear
	Foot care education
	Avoid walking bare foot
	Use of light color socks
	Referral to podiatrist
	Mobility assistive devices (eg, cane, walker)
	Physical therapy
Vision impairment	Visual aids (use of mirrors for better visualization of feet)
Chronic pain	Adequate pain management

Data from Refs.[25,28,40–42]

Type 1 Diabetes Mellitus

Insulin therapy is required for people with type 1 diabetes. Strategies for insulin delivery differ between healthy older adults and those with frailty and limited life expectancy.[43] Family members and caretakers should also receive diabetes education, including training in the administration of insulin and glucagon and in the use of self-monitoring of blood glucose (SMBG). Frequent SMBG is important to guide insulin therapy and detect and avoid hypoglycemia. The use of continuous glucose monitoring systems (CGMS) may also be helpful.

Type 1 diabetes treatment requires multiple insulin injections daily or use of an insulin pump. Over time, these complex insulin regimens can become difficult for a frail older patient to manage. If assistance in insulin administration is unavailable, insulin regimens may need to be simplified according to the patient's ability and preferences to minimize errors.[44]

Injection (basal-bolus) therapy

- In both older and younger adults, injection therapy usually combines a long-acting basal insulin analog (commonly once-daily insulin glargine or once-daily or twice-daily insulin detemir) and a rapidly acting insulin analog for boluses (commonly insulin aspart, lispro, or glulisine) with meals.
- If the patient cannot afford to purchase the more expensive long-acting basal insulin analogs (glargine or detemir), intermediate-acting NPH (neutral protamine Hagedorn) insulin can be given before breakfast and at bedtime. Use of NPH insulin is associated with increased risk for hypoglycemia if the lunch meal is missed. Snacks may be needed mid morning, mid afternoon, and at bedtime to avoid hypoglycemia.[45,46] Glucose levels should be occasionally checked in the middle of the night to exclude nocturnal hypoglycemia.
- Basal insulin should not be withheld during intercurrent illness or during periods of poor oral intake, because this could lead to severe hyperglycemia and diabetic ketoacidosis.
- Prandial insulin dosing is based on the premeal blood glucose level and anticipated carbohydrate intake for that particular meal. Calculations commonly use a correction (sensitivity) factor to decrease glucose to desired target level and insulin/carbohydrate ratios (or fixed dosing for fixed carbohydrate content of meals) to determine mealtime doses. This approach becomes more difficult with cognitive decline.[44] Calculators (eg, apps for smart phones and built into insulin pumps) are available.
- If there is unreliable food intake, rapidly acting insulin analogs (lispro, aspart, or glulisine) can be given immediately after the meal so that a lower dose can be given if less food (carbohydrate) was ingested.
- If rapidly acting insulin analogs cannot be purchased, less expensive regular insulin can be used before meals. This insulin has a slower onset and longer duration of action, so it is more likely to cause hypoglycemia several hours after the meal. Snacks may be needed mid to late morning and afternoon and at bedtime. If regular insulin is used with NPH insulin, a lunchtime dose of regular insulin may not be needed.
- Rarely, NPH and regular insulin are used twice daily (before breakfast and dinner).[47,48] This regimen may be used if the patient has difficulty with self-administration of insulin and assistance is not available at lunch and bedtime. Premixed insulins are rarely used in type 1 diabetes, because of their nonphysiologic profiles and lack of flexibility to match mealtime requirements.

- Insulin pens, magnifiers for insulin syringes, and other aids are available for individuals with impaired vision, hearing, and dexterity (see **Table 3**).

Insulin pump/continuous subcutaneous insulin infusion therapy

- A rapidly acting insulin analog (lispro, aspart or glulisine) is delivered continuously to provide basal requirements; boluses are delivered for meals and to correct hyperglycemia. Infusion sets are changed every 2 to 3 days.
- Continuous subcutaneous insulin infusion (CSII) has not been studied extensively in the elderly population, but preliminary studies suggest that it may improve glycemic control and reduce hypoglycemia to the same extent in patients aged between 50 and 65 years as it does in younger patients. Experts routinely recommend continuing CSII in patients who continue to be appropriate candidates.[49]
- Advantages of CSII include the ability to program multiple basal rates, the ability to use reduced temporary basal rates for increased activity, and availability of an insulin bolus calculator (incorporated into the pump) to calculate bolus dosing based on the glucose level and carbohydrate intake.[49]
- As older adults experience functional or cognitive decline, the use of CSII may become difficult. CSII therapy can be continued if the individual (or their partner/caregivers) has received the appropriate training and is capable of properly operating the pump.

Continuous glucose monitoring systems

- Sensors measure glucose levels in the interstitial fluid. Calibration with SMBG is required.
- CGMS alerts individuals when glucose levels increase higher than or decrease lower than preset glucose levels to help avoid serious hyperglycemic/hypoglycemic episodes.
- CGMS is particularly useful in adults with wide glycemic excursions, poor hypoglycemia awareness, or a history of serious hypoglycemia.
- The use of a CGMS-augmented insulin pump with a low glucose threshold suspend feature (suspending insulin infusion for ≤ 2 hours in the presence of hypoglycemia) helps reduce serious hypoglycemia without deterioration in A_{1c} level.[50] This strategy may be particularly helpful in older adults, given their high risk of hypoglycemia, but further studies in the elderly are needed.

Type 2 Diabetes

For most older adults with type 2 diabetes, initial pharmacologic treatment is an oral medication. The choice of initial therapy is guided by safety, tolerability, hypoglycemia risk, cost, ease of administration, renal and hepatic status, and patient preference. Combination oral therapy may be needed. Available noninsulin therapies and associated side effects are summarized in **Table 4**. Insulin is added when oral therapy is insufficient to maintain glycemic goals.

- Low-dose metformin is generally the preferred first line of treatment in older adults. It should be avoided in patients 80 years of age or older in the presence of impaired renal function and higher doses (eg, >1000 mg/d) should be used cautiously.
- Glipizide is the preferred sulfonylurea in the elderly, because it is the least dependent on renal function for excretion and is associated with less hypoglycemia

Table 4
Oral and noninsulin injectable medications for the treatment of type 2 diabetes in the elderly

Medication	Primary Mechanism of Action	Geriatric Dosing	Most Common Side Effects	Geriatric Considerations	Generic Available
Metformin (Glucophage, Glumetza, Fortamet)	Decreases hepatic glucose production	Initial dose: 500 mg daily. Maintenance dose: 500 mg twice daily or 850 mg once daily Use higher doses cautiously	Diarrhea, abdominal discomfort, constipation, dyspepsia (these GI effects can be transient) Also anorexia, metallic taste, decreased vitamin B_{12}	Use with caution in patients >80 y with careful adherence to recommended renal dose adjustments. Do not use if eGFR<30 mL/ min/1.73 m² If eGFR 30–45 mL/min/ 1.73 m², use maximum 1000 mg daily	Yes
Sulfonylureas Glimepiride (Amaryl) Glipizide (Glucotrol) Glyburide (Diabeta, Glynase)	Stimulate insulin release from the pancreas	Glimepiride: initial dose: 0.5–1 mg once daily Glipizide: immediate release tablet: 2.5 mg once daily For both, glimepiride and glipizide, dose titration and maintenance dose should be conservative to avoid hypoglycemia (not to exceed 50% of maximum dose)	Hypoglycemia	Avoid long-acting sulfonylureas (especially glyburide) because of the risk of prolonged hypoglycemia Drug excretion of glipizide is least dependent on renal function Glipizide is the preferred sulfonylurea in elderly (least hypoglycemia) Glyburide is not preferred in elderly, because of increased risk of hypoglycemia and weight gain	Yes

Drug class / Agents	Mechanism	Dosing	Adverse effects	Cautions	
Meglitinides Repaglinide (Prandin) Nateglinide (Starlix)	Stimulate glucose-dependent insulin release from the pancreatic β cells	Repaglinide: flexible meal dosing; titrate dose cautiously. Patients not previously treated or whose HbA_{1c} is <8%: initial dose 0.5 mg before each meal. Patients previously treated with blood glucose-lowering agents whose HbA_{1c} is ≥8%: 1 mg before each meal. Nateglinide: 60 mg 3 times daily before meals	Hypoglycemia	Use with caution because of risk of hypoglycemia	Yes
Thiazolidinediones Pioglitazone (Actos) Rosiglitazone (Avandia)	Peroxisome proliferator-activated receptor γ agonists; improve insulin sensitivity in adipose tissue, liver, and skeletal muscle	Pioglitazone: 15 mg once daily. Rosiglitazone: 2–4 mg daily as a single daily dose or in divided doses twice daily	Edema, heart failure, weight gain, fractures, increased risk of bladder cancer (pioglitazone)	Avoid in elderly because of increased fluid retention, exacerbation of heart failure and increased risk of fractures. Not recommended in patients with symptomatic heart failure	Pioglitazone: yes
α-Glucosidase inhibitors Acarbose (Precose) Miglitol (Glyset)	Intestinal α-glucosidase inhibitors; delay intestinal absorption of glucose	25 mg 3 times daily at the start of each meal	Diarrhea, flatulence, abdominal pain	Not recommended if CrCl ≤24 mL/min. GI side effects limit use	Acarbose: yes

(continued on next page)

Table 4
(continued)

Medication	Primary Mechanism of Action	Geriatric Dosing	Most Common Side Effects	Geriatric Considerations	Generic Available
DPP-4 inhibitors Sitagliptin (Januvia) Saxagliptin (Onglyza) Linagliptin (Tradjenta) Alogliptin (Nesina)	Inhibit DPP-4, resulting in prolonged action of GLP-1 (increase insulin release, reduce glucagon secretion)	Sitagliptin: 100 mg once daily CrCl 30–50 mL/min: 50 mg once daily CrCl <30 mL/min: 25 mg once daily Saxagliptin: 2.5–5.0 mg once daily For CrCl ≤50 mL/min: 2.5 mg once daily Linagliptin: 5 mg once daily Alogliptin: 25 mg once daily CrCl 30–50 mL/min: 12.5 mg once daily CrCl <30 mL/min: 6.25 mg once daily	Possible pancreatitis Possible increased risk of heart failure outcomes Unknown long-term side effects	Dose should be adjusted for renal impairment, except linagliptin	No
GLP-1 receptor agonists Exenatide (Byetta, Bydureon) Liraglutide (Victoza) Albiglutide (Tanzeum) Dulaglutide (Trulicity)	Increase glucose-dependent insulin secretion, decrease inappropriate glucagon secretion, slow gastric emptying, and increase satiety	*Exenatide:* Immediate release (Byetta): Initial: 5 µg subcut twice daily within 60 min before a meal; after 1 mo, may be increased to 10 µg twice daily (based on response) Extended release (Bydureon): 2 mg subcut once weekly Liraglutide: 0.6 mg subcut once daily for 1 wk; then increase to 1.2 mg once daily; may increase further to 1.8 mg once daily if optimal glycemic response not achieved with 1.2 mg/d Albiglutide: 30 mg subcut once weekly Dulaglutide: 0.75 mg once weekly; maximum 1.5 mg weekly	Hypoglycemia (in combination therapy with sulfonylurea or insulin), nausea (dose-dependent), vomiting, diarrhea, constipation, dyspepsia, weight loss, possible pancreatitis	Injectable Few studies in older adults	No

Drug	Mechanism of action	Dosing	Adverse effects	Considerations in the elderly	Renal dose adjustment
SGLT2 inhibitors Canagliflozin (Invokana) Dapagliflozin (Farxiga) Empagliflozin (Jardiance)	Inhibit SGLT2 in the proximal renal tubules, reduce glucose reabsorption, lower renal threshold for glucose, resulting in increased urinary excretion of glucose	Canagliflozin: 100 mg once daily before first meal of the day Do not use if eGFR <45 mL/min/1.73 m^2 Dapagliflozin: 5 mg once daily in the morning, with or without food Do not use if eGFR <60 mL/min/1.73 m^2 Empagliflozin: 10 mg once daily Do not use if eGFR <45 mL/min/1.73 m^2	Renal insufficiency, hypovolemia, hypotension, syncope, dehydration, genital mycotic infections, UTIs, polyuria, worsened urinary incontinence	Elderly patients may be predisposed to intravascular volume depletion (hypotension, orthostatic hypotension, dizziness, syncope, and dehydration), renal impairment or failure, increased genital mycotic and urinary infections, and worsened urinary incontinence HbA$_{1c}$ reductions may be lower in patients >65 y compared with younger patients	No
Amylin agonist Pramlintide (Symlin)	Delays gastric emptying and inhibits the release of glucagon, reducing the rate of glucose absorption	15 µg subcut immediately before major meal, increased by 15 µg every 3–7 d as tolerated	Nausea, vomiting, abdominal pain, anorexia	Increased risk of severe hypoglycemia in elderly with concomitant use of insulin Avoid use in elderly	No

Abbreviations: CrCl, creatinine clearance; DPP-4, dipeptidyl peptidase 4; GI, gastrointestinal; GLP-1, glucagonlike peptide 1; HbA$_{1c}$, hemoglobin A$_{1c}$; SGLT2, sodium-glucose cotransporter 2; UTI, urinary tract infection.
Data from Refs.[51–53]

than the longer-acting sulfonylurea drugs. Glyburide should not be used because of a higher risk of hypoglycemia.

- Dipeptidyl peptidase 4 (DPP-4) inhibitors are safe, weight neutral, and well tolerated in the elderly but are more expensive than metformin or glipizide. Increased rate of heart failure outcomes is possible.[54] The dose of linagliptin does not need to be changed with declining renal function.

- Meglitinides are short acting and allow for flexible meal dosing but need to be given with each meal and used cautiously. They primarily decrease postprandial blood glucose levels. Hypoglycemia is a potential risk, but this risk is lower than with sulfonylurea drugs.[55]

- Thiazolidinediones cause fluid retention and are associated with weight gain and worsening of heart failure. There is also increased risk of fracture. Pioglitazone is associated with increased risk of bladder cancer. These drugs are generally not recommended in the elderly.

- α-Glucosidase inhibitors delay the absorption of glucose, reducing postprandial glycemic levels.[56] They are associated with gastrointestinal side effects (especially flatulence and diarrhea) and need to be taken with each meal, which can be difficult in the elderly.

- Glucagonlike peptide 1 receptor agonists are injectable and can cause nausea, vomiting, and weight loss. These effects could be problematic in the frail and malnourished elderly.[48,57] They have not been well studied in older adults and are generally not recommended in this population.

- Sodium-glucose cotransporter 2 inhibitors can predispose the elderly to intravascular volume depletion and decline in renal function and increases the risk of genital mycotic infections.[48,58] There can be worsening of urinary incontinence, weight loss, and more urinary tract infections in older women.

- Insulin therapy is indicated when monotherapy or combined therapy with oral medications fails to achieve the desired glycemic target.[46,47] Insulin should be introduced at low dose only if needed and with caution in the elderly.[59,60] A basal insulin analog (insulin glargine or detemir) can be added to oral regimens in the presence of fasting hyperglycemia. Care is needed not to give too much basal insulin; fasting glucose levels can reflect not only basal needs but evening food intake. Hypoglycemia is a significant risk.

- If postprandial hyperglycemia is the main cause of an increased A_{1c} level, a rapidly acting insulin analog (insulin aspart, lispro, glulisine) can be added to the largest meal(s) rather than initiating basal insulin. If there is unreliable food intake, the rapidly acting insulin analog can be given immediately after the meal so that a lower dose can be given if less food (carbohydrate) is ingested. Elderly patients with renal insufficiency may experience fewer hypoglycemic episodes when using rapidly acting insulin analogs (compared with longer-acting insulins).[44,59]

- If basal-bolus insulin injection therapy is needed, recommendations are similar to those described earlier for the management of type 1 diabetes.

- Insulin administration using vials and syringes can be difficult for the elderly, who may have vision impairment and declining manual dexterity. The use of prefilled insulin pens and other aids can be helpful.[61]

NONPHARMACOLOGIC STRATEGIES

Diabetes self-management education and training (DSME/T) is essential and should involve the patient, caregivers, family and friends. DSME/T includes instructions concerning monitoring, medical nutrition therapy, proper administration of medications, sick day rules, and physical activity guidelines. Blood glucose awareness training can also be useful for people with poor hypoglycemic awareness. The American Diabetes Association publishes a consumer guide to diabetes-related products annually in *Diabetes Forecast*.

SMBG frequency should be individualized. For those with satisfactory and stable glycemic control taking oral drugs not associated with hypoglycemia, infrequent testing (0–2 times daily) is reasonable. Medicare Part B covers 100 glucose monitoring strips every 3 months for patients not receiving insulin. Adults on insulin therapy should test more frequently (2–6 times daily), depending on the insulin regimen and propensity for hypoglycemia. For those using a basal-bolus insulin regimen, SMBG should be performed before meals, bedtime, and as needed (eg, with signs or symptoms of hypoglycemia, before driving, before and after exercise, and in the middle of the night for evaluation of nocturnal hypoglycemia). Medicare Part B pays for 300 strips every 3 months for individuals taking insulin, but additional strips can be requested if the treating physician states that they are medically necessary.

Recommendations should be communicated in simple terms aided by visual handouts, models, and written instructions. Addressing barriers such as vision and hearing impairments, pain control, transportation difficulties, caregiver stress, difficulty swallowing, cognitive decline, depression, and problems obtaining or administering medications are important.[41] Nutrition therapy combined with physical activity can improve glycemic and blood pressure control, help preserve, improve, or slow decline in function, and reduce cardiometabolic risk in older adults.[46]

Medical Nutrition Therapy

Medical nutrition therapy is an essential component of diabetes care. In the geriatric population, general nutrition concerns as well as diabetes-specific issues should be addressed. Older adults are at risk for malnutrition, including micronutrient deficiencies caused by anorexia, altered taste and smell, swallowing difficulties, and oral/dental issues. Functional impairments leading to difficulties in preparing or consuming food result in dependence on others for meals and shopping and other medical comorbidities.[62,63] Weight loss, whether intentional or unintentional, may contribute to nutritional deficits and worsen sarcopenia. Fortified foods and nutritional supplements, including vitamins and minerals, may be needed.

For the older adult with diabetes, specific dietary recommendations can vary, depending on their general nutritional status, and whether the individual requires insulin therapy. For those who require basal-bolus insulin therapy (eg, those with type 1 diabetes), mealtime insulin dosing should primarily match the carbohydrate content of meals. This regimen can be especially challenging in elderly patients with inconsistent food intake or poor numeracy skills. Errors can cause wide glycemic fluctuations. In the presence of poor and unpredictable food intake, the use of carbohydrate-consistent meals may be helpful, and consideration should be given to administering rapid-acting insulin immediately after meals, so lower doses can be given if less food is consumed.[64]

The diet should be individualized to conform to the patient's lifestyle, food preferences, nutritional needs, and socioeconomic factors. Changes may need to be introduced gradually to enhance adherence.[63,65,66] Adults with type 1 diabetes may also have celiac disease, further affecting food choices. Interventions such as providing small, frequent meals, fortified food, protein shakes, dysphagia diet, or formula feed can also improve caloric intake when needed.[28] A healthy balanced low-salt diet containing complex carbohydrates and fiber, particularly fruits and vegetables, lean proteins, and less than 20% total fat can help improve glycemic and blood pressure control and reduce the need for medications. Older adults may find community resources such as Meals on Wheels or meals served at local senior centers beneficial.[28]

Physical Activity

Engaging in regular physical activity is an integral part of diabetes care. Older adults with diabetes who are otherwise healthy and functional (youthful older adults) should be encouraged to engage in aerobic activity for 150 min/wk or more. If the individual has been sedentary, this activity may need to be gradually introduced. Those with known heart disease or multiple cardiovascular risk factors, osteoarthritis, chronic lung disease, osteoporosis, or other serious comorbidities should have exercise recommendations revised appropriately. Cardiac testing may be recommended. Exercise regimes should be individualized according to need, functional status, presence of comorbidities, geriatric syndromes, and age.

Muscle mass and strength decline with age, presence of comorbidities, malnutrition, and periods of prolonged immobilization and hospitalization. Physical and occupational therapy can be useful. Fall prevention is critical. Exercise programs prescribed by specialized physical trainers take into account the physical and psychological capabilities of the older adult.[46] Joining supervised group exercise programs at senior centers, YMCAs, and other community facilities can also be of benefit.

For adults using insulin therapy or taking insulin secretagogues, physical activity can cause hypoglycemia. Instructions on ways to avoid hypoglycemia (reduced medication dosing or eating snacks) and treat hypoglycemia should be provided. It is important to convey that hypoglycemia can occur not only during activity but for a prolonged period after the activity. Glucose monitoring should be used. Wearing a medical alert bracelet or necklace and use of Medical Alert services (eg, pendant or watch medical alert alarm monitoring systems) can be life saving.

EVALUATION AND ADJUSTMENT

The management of diabetes in the elderly includes ongoing individualized assessments, with modifications in the treatment plan as indicated. Periodic assessments for geriatric syndromes (physical function, nutrition, cognition, comorbidities, depression, polypharmacy, pain, incontinence, social support) are recommended. Glycemic, blood pressure, and lipid goals change over time. Elements of routine follow-up diabetes care in the elderly are outlined later.

Screening for diabetes-related complications is also an integral part of diabetes care. For relatively healthy older adults, the screening examinations described later are recommended. For the frail elderly or those with multiple comorbidities and short life expectancy, it is reasonable to consider the expected benefit, burden of intervening, and patient preference.

Diabetes Self-Management Education and Training

The importance of periodic diabetes education, including nutrition counseling, has been previously described. In general, Medicare Part B (medical insurance) pays for 10 hours of initial training and an additional 2 hours annually (exclusive of medical nutrition therapy) if prescribed by a physician and obtained in a program certified by the American Diabetes Association or the Indian Health Service. Medical nutrition therapy is covered if delivered by a registered dietitian or certain other nutrition professionals.

Glycemic Control

Glycemic goals, control, and treatment plans should be reevaluated using A_{1c} testing, review of SMBG logs, consideration of the presence or progression of geriatric syndromes and comorbidities, and history of hypoglycemia. It is important to avoid overtreatment, especially in those with limited life expectancy, frailty, low GFR, and moderate to severe cognitive impairment or dementia. Frequent communications or visits may be needed.[67,68]

Blood Pressure Control

Blood pressure should be measured at each medical visit, and goals and medications reevaluated. Home blood pressure monitoring may be helpful.

Lipid Management

A lipid profile should be checked annually and statin medications prescribed (if tolerated) in those with CVD or at least 1 additional risk factor (hypertension, smoking, dyslipidemia, albuminuria, or family history of CVD) in the absence of a limited life expectancy.[38] As discussed earlier, use of statin drugs in adults older than 80 years or with major comorbidities is controversial. The benefits of fenofibrate for those older than 65 years with mild to moderate hypertriglyceridemia have not been established.[69]

Eye Care

Eye examinations should be performed annually or as recommended by the eye care specialist. Screening for diabetic retinopathy and macular edema as well as for glaucoma should be performed. Cataracts are also more common in diabetes. If there is impaired vision, appropriate evaluation, treatment, and correction for refractive errors or recommendations for vision aids can improve quality of life and help prevent errors in medication administration.

Foot Care

Examination of the feet should occur at each medical visit. Referral to a podiatrist should be considered in the presence of foot deformities, neuropathy, peripheral vascular disease, or a history of foot ulcers or other foot disease. Caregivers should be involved in regular inspection of feet, nail clipping (if the patient is incapable and is not receiving this service from a provider), and proper cleaning of feet when necessary. Proper fitting shoes and white socks (for easy visibility of blood stains) are recommended.

Medicare Part B pays for 1 pair of therapeutic shoes and inserts each year if (1) the physician treating the diabetes certifies that they are needed (presence of $\geq$1 of the following: amputation, history of foot ulcer, peripheral vascular disease, foot deformities, neuropathy with callus, or preulcerative callus) and (2) the shoes/inserts are prescribed by a podiatrist or other qualified doctor. Further details are available at http://www.medicare.gov.

Renal Function

Monitoring renal function (serum creatinine and eGFR) in the elderly is important, because decline in renal function is common and necessitates adjustments of medications. In healthy older adults, annual screening for albuminuria, with treatment with an ACE-I or ARB in the presence of persistent microalbuminuria, should be considered. ACE-I and ARBs should not be used in combination.[70]

Additional Recommendations

- Smoking status should be assessed and cessation recommended.
- Aspirin (75–162 mg), if tolerated and not contraindicated, should be considered in the presence of CVD or at least 1 additional risk factor (hypertension, smoking, dyslipidemia, albuminuria, or family history of CVD).[71] Because the elderly are at increased risk of bleeding, potential benefit versus risk must be carefully considered.
- Concerns about social support and financial resources should be elicited, with referral to a social worker or other resources as needed.
- In obese older adults with symptoms suggestive of sleep apnea, screening should be considered.
- Periodontal disease is more common in diabetes. Dental problems can adversely affect eating/nutrition. Consideration should be given for dental care referral.
- The immunization history should be reviewed, and annual influenza vaccination administered. Pneumonia and shingles vaccine should also be offered as per standard vaccination guidelines.[72,73]

FUTURE CONSIDERATIONS/SUMMARY

With the increasing prevalence of diabetes in the elderly, better management approaches to meet the unique needs of this growing population are needed. This strategy includes more research on the optimal use of oral glycemic control medications in the elderly, better aids to assist individuals with impairments in vision, cognition, and mobility, and safer methods of insulin administration to avoid hypoglycemia. Progress in the development of CGMS, new glycemic control agents, and advances in the development of an artificial pancreas also hold great promise.

Diverse methods of delivering diabetes care to the elderly have been investigated. The use of group visits[74] and team care, with interim phone contact,[41,75] can be helpful. Telemedicine has been shown to be of benefit in several studies.[76] The Informatics for Diabetes and Education Telemedicine (IDEATel) demonstration project in ethnically diverse Medicare beneficiaries used nurse educators and dietitians to conduct home televisits every 6 weeks or as needed. During televisits, self-management education was provided, downloads of home blood glucose and blood pressure values, and annual laboratory data were reviewed, and under the supervision of endocrinologists, recommendations for changes in treatment were made to primary care providers. This project resulted in better glycemic, blood pressure, and lipid control and reduced disparities.[77–79] Participation in the telemedicine intervention was also associated with lessened decline in physical activity, impairment, and cognition.[80,81] In addition, we have shown in a pilot study in a long-term care facility that review of glucose values and medications by an endocrinologist using telemedicine has the potential to improve glycemia, including reduction of hypoglycemia.[82] Additional investigation in this area is needed.

Until results of further research in the elderly with diabetes become available, it is important to individualize, assess, and adjust diabetes care plans periodically with input from the patient and their caretakers. The development or advancement of geriatric syndromes, hypoglycemia, and comorbidities will direct the need for further diabetes education and training, additional social services, and modification of pharmacologic therapy. When possible, use of medications with low risk for hypoglycemia (eg, metformin, DPP-4 inhibitors) is advisable. Initial therapy should use low doses; insulin must be used with caution. Goals should include minimizing hypoglycemia, symptomatic hyperglycemia, orthostatic hypotension, and other drug-related complications and maintaining quality of life.

REFERENCES

1. US Centers for Disease Control and Prevention: National Diabetes Statistics Report, 2014. Available at: http://www.cdc.gov/diabetes/pubs/statsreport14.htm. Accessed June 20, 2014.
2. Selvin E, Parrinello CM, Sacks DB, et al. Trends in prevalence and control of diabetes in the United States, 1988-1994 and 1999-2010. Ann Intern Med 2014; 160(8):517–25.
3. Andreassen LM, Sandberg S, Kristensen GB, et al. Nursing home patients with diabetes: prevalence, drug treatment and glycemic control. Diabetes Res Clin Pract 2014;105(1):102–9.
4. Gregg EW, Beckles GL, Williamson DF, et al. Diabetes and physical disability among older US adults. Diabetes Care 2000;23(9):1272–7.
5. Gregg EW, Li Y, Wang J, et al. Changes in diabetes related complications in the United States, 1990-2010. N Engl J Med 2014;370(16):1514–23.
6. Currie CJ, Peters JR, Tynan A, et al. Survival as a function of HbA1c in people with type 2 diabetes: a retrospective cohort study. Lancet 2010;375(9713):481–9.
7. Huang ES, Liu JY, Moffet HH, et al. Glycemic control, complications, and death in older diabetic patients: the diabetes and aging study. Diabetes Care 2011;34(6): 1329–36.
8. Sanon VP, Sanon S, Kanakia R, et al. Hypoglycemia from a cardiologist's perspective. Clin Cardiol 2014. http://dx.doi.org/10.1002/clc.22288. Available at: http://www.ncbi.nlm.nih.gov/pubmed?term=Chilton%20R%5BAuthor%5D&cauthor=true&cauthor_uid=24895268.
9. Tseng CL, Soroka O, Maney M, et al. Asssessing potential glycemic overtreatment in persons at hypoglycemic risk. JAMA Intern Med 2014;174(2):259–68.
10. Lipska KJ, Ross JS, Wang Y, et al. National trends in US hospital admissions for hyperglycemia and hypoglycemia among Medicare beneficiaries, 1999 to 2011. JAMA Intern Med 2014;174(7):1116–24.
11. Geller AI, Shehab N, Lovegrove MC, et al. National estimates of insulin-related hypoglycemia and errors leading to emergency department visits and hospitalizations. JAMA Intern Med 2014;174(5):678–86.
12. Majumdar SR, Hemmelgarn BR, Lin M, et al. Hypoglycemia associated with hospitalization and adverse events in older people: population-based cohort study. Diabetes Care 2013;36(11):3585–90.
13. Weinstock RS, Xing D, Maahs DM, et al. T1D Exchange Clinic Network. Severe hypoglycemia and diabetic ketoacidosis in adults with type 1 diabetes: results from the T1D Exchange clinic registry. J Clin Endocrinol Metab 2013;98(8): 3411–9.
14. Gold AE, Macleod KM, Frier BM. Frequency of severe hypoglycemia in patients with type 1 diabetes with impaired awareness of hypoglycemia. Diabetes Care 1994;17(7):697–703.
15. Matyka K, Evans M, Lomas J, et al. Altered hierarchy of protective responses against severe hypoglycemia in normal aging in healthy men. Diabetes Care 1997;20(2):135–41.
16. Brierley EJ, Broughton DL, James OF, et al. Reduced awareness of hypoglycaemia in the elderly despite an intact counter-regulatory response. Q J Med 1995; 88(6):439–45.
17. Bremer JP, Jauch-Chara K, Hallschmid M, et al. Hypoglycemia unawareness in older compared with middle-aged patients with type 2 diabetes. Diabetes Care 2009;32(8):1513–7.

18. Cryer PE. Hypoglycemia in type 1 diabetes mellitus. Endocrinol Metab Clin North Am 2010;39(3):641–54.
19. Whitmer RA, Karter AJ, Yaffe K, et al. Hypoglycemic episodes and risk of dementia in older patients with type 2 diabetes mellitus. JAMA 2009;301(15): 1565–72.
20. Feinkohl I, Aung PP, Keller M, et al. Severe hypoglycemia and cognitive decline in older people with type 2 diabetes: the Edinburgh Type 2 Diabetes Study. Diabetes Care 2014;37(2):507–15.
21. Nordin C. The case for hypoglycaemia as a proarrhythmic event: basic and clinical evidence. Diabetologia 2010;53(8):1552–61.
22. Bonds DE, Miller ME, Bergenstal RM, et al. The association between symptomatic, severe hypoglycaemia and mortality in type 2 diabetes: retrospective epidemiological analysis of the ACCORD study. BMJ 2010;340:b4909.
23. Zoungas S, Patel A, Chalmers J, et al, ADVANCE Collaborative Group. Severe hypoglycemia and risks of vascular events and death. N Engl J Med 2010;363(15): 1410–8.
24. Green AJ, Fox KM, Grandy S, SHIELD Study Group. Self-reported hypoglycemia and impact on quality of life and depression among adults with type 2 diabetes mellitus. Diabetes Res Clin Pract 2012;96(3):313–8.
25. Trief P, Xing D, Foster N, et al. Depression in adults in the T1D exchange clinic registry. Depression in adults in the T1D exchange clinic registry. Diabetes Care 2014;37(6):1563–72.
26. Laiteerapong N, Karter AJ, Liu JY, et al. Correlates of quality of life in older adults with diabetes: the Diabetes & Aging Study. Diabetes Care 2011;34(8):1749–53.
27. Araki A, Ito H. Diabetes mellitus and geriatric syndromes. Geriatr Gerontol Int 2009;9(2):105–14.
28. Kirkman MS, Briscoe VJ, Clark N, et al. Consensus Development Conference on Diabetes and Older Adults. Diabetes in older adults: a consensus report. J Am Geriatr Soc 2012;60(12):2342–56.
29. Rydén L, Grant PJ, Anker SD, et al. ESC Guidelines on diabetes, pre-diabetes, and cardiovascular diseases developed in collaboration with the EASD: the Task Force on diabetes, pre-diabetes, and cardiovascular diseases of the European Society of Cardiology (ESC) and developed in collaboration with the European Association for the Study of Diabetes (EASD). Eur Heart J 2013;34(39): 3035–87.
30. International Diabetes Federation Global Guideline for Managing Older People with Type 2 Diabetes. 2013. Available at: http://www.idf.org/guidelines/managing-older-people-type-2-diabetes. Accessed June 12, 2014.
31. Sinclair A, Morley JE, Rodriguez-Manas L, et al. Diabetes mellitus in older people: position statement on behalf of the International Association of Gerontology and Geriatrics (IAGG), the European Diabetes Working Party for Older People (EDWPOP), and the International Task Force of Experts in Diabetes. J Am Med Dir Assoc 2012;13(6):497–502.
32. The Department of Veterans Affairs and the Department of Defense Clinical Practice Guidelines. Management of diabetes in primary care. 2010. Available at: http://www.healthquality.va.gov/guidelines/CD/diabetes/DM2010_FUL-v4e.pdf. Accessed July 1, 2014.
33. The Department of Veterans Affairs and the Department of Defense Clinical Practice Guidelines. Management of hypertension in primary care. 2005. Available at: http://www.healthquality.va.gov/guidelines/CD/htn/htn04_pdf1.pdf. Accessed July 1, 2014.

34. The Department of Veterans Affairs and the Department of Defense Clinical Practice Guidelines. Management of dyslipidemia. 2006. Available at: http://www.healthquality.va.gov/guidelines/CD/lipids/lip05_950_final2.pdf. Accessed July 1, 2014.
35. James PA, Oparil S, Carter BL, et al. 2014 evidence-based guideline for the management of high blood pressure in adults: report from the panel members appointed to the Eighth Joint National Committee (JNC 8). JAMA 2014;13(5):507–20.
36. Mancia G, Fagard R, Narkiewicz K, et al. 2013 ESH/ESC guidelines for the management of arterial hypertension. Blood Press 2014;23(1):3–16.
37. Stone NJ, Robinson J, Lichtenstein AH, et al. 2013 ACC/AHA guideline on the treatment of blood cholesterol to reduce atherosclerotic cardiovascular risk in adults: a report of the American College of Cardiology/American Heart Association Task Force on Practice Guidelines. Circulation 2014;129(25Suppl 2):S1–45.
38. Solano MP, Goldberg RB. Management of dyslipidemia in diabetes. Cardiol Rev 2006;14(3):125–35.
39. Petersen LK, Christensen K, Kragstrup J. Lipid-lowering treatment to the end? A review of observational studies and RCTs on cholesterol and mortality in 80+-year-olds. Age Ageing 2010;39(6):674–80.
40. American Geriatrics Society 2012 Beers Criteria Update Expert Panel. American Geriatrics Society updated Beers Criteria for potentially inappropriate medication use in older adults. J Am Geriatr Soc 2012;60(4):616–31.
41. Munshi MN, Segal AR, Suhl E, et al. Assessment of barriers to improve diabetes management in older adults. Diabetes Care 2013;36(3):543–9.
42. Aids for insulin users 2014. Diabetes Forecast. Available at: http://www.diabetesforecast.org/2014/Jan/aids-for-insulin-users-2014.html. Accessed July 06, 2014.
43. Dhaliwal R, Weinstock RS. Management of type 1 diabetes in older adults. Diabetes Spectr 2014;27(1):9–20.
44. Ober SK, Watts S, Lawrence RH. Insulin use in elderly diabetic patients. Clin Interv Aging 2006;1(2):107–13.
45. Ligthelm RJ, Kaiser M, Vora J, et al. Insulin use in elderly adults: risk of hypoglycemia and strategies for care. J Am Geriatr Soc 2012;60(8):1564–70.
46. Rosenstock J. Management of type 2 diabetes mellitus in the elderly. Drugs Aging 2001;18(1):31–44.
47. Hendra TJ. Starting insulin therapy in elderly patients. J R Soc Med 2002;95(9):453–5.
48. Drugs for type 2 diabetes. Treat Guidel Med Lett 2014;12(139):17–24. Available at: http://www.medicalletter.org.
49. Matejko B, Cyganek K, Katra B, et al. Insulin pump therapy is equally effective and safe in elderly and young type 1 diabetes patients. Rev Diabet Stud 2011;8(2):254–8.
50. Bergenstal RM, Klonoff DC, Garg SK, et al, ASPIRE In-Home Study Group. Threshold-based insulin pump interruption for reduction of hypoglycemia. N Engl J Med 2013;369(3):224–32.
51. Lipska KJ, Bailey CJ, Inzucchi SE. Use of metformin in the setting of mild-to-moderate renal insufficiency. Diabetes Care 2011;34(6):1431–7.
52. Riddle MC. More reasons to say goodbye to glyburide. J Clin Endocrinol Metab 2010;95(11):4867–70.
53. Round EM, Engel SS, Golm GT, et al. Safety and tolerability of sitagliptin in elderly patients with type 2 diabetes: a pooled analysis of 25 clinical studies. Drugs Aging 2014;31(3):203–14.

54. Wu S, Hopper I, Skip M, et al. Dipeptidyl peptidase-4 inhibitors and cardiovascular outcomes: meta-analysis of randomized clinical trials with 55,141 participants. Cardiovasc Ther 2014;32(4):147–58. http://dx.doi.org/10.1111/1755-5922.12075.

55. Plosker GL, Figgitt DP. Repaglinide: a pharmacoeconomic review of its use in type 2 diabetes mellitus. Pharmacoeconomics 2004;22(6):389–411.

56. van de Laar FA, Lucassen PL, Akkermans RP, et al. Alpha-glucosidase inhibitors for patients with type 2 diabetes: results from a Cochrane systematic review and meta-analysis. Diabetes Care 2005;28(1):154–63.

57. Miller EM. Individualizing care with injectable glucose-lowering agents. J Fam Pract 2013;62(12 Suppl CME):S12–9.

58. Ferrannini E, Solini A. SGLT2 inhibition in diabetes mellitus: rationale and clinical prospects. Nat Rev Endocrinol 2012;8(8):495–502.

59. Sharma V, Aggarwal S, Sharma A. Diabetes in elderly. J Endocrinol Metab 2011; 1(1):9–13.

60. Odegard PS, Setter SM, Neumiller JJ. Considerations for the pharmacological treatment of diabetes in older adults. Diabetes Spectr 2007;20(4):239–47.

61. Lostia S, Lunetta M, Lunetta M, et al. Safety, efficacy, acceptability of a pre-filled insulin pen in diabetic patients over 60 years old. Diabetes Res Clin Pract 1995; 28(3):173–7.

62. Sullivan DH, Bopp MM, Roberson PK. Protein-energy undernutrition and life-threatening complications among the hospitalized elderly. J Gen Intern Med 2002;17(12):923–32.

63. Wells JL, Dumbrell AC. Nutrition and aging: assessment and treatment of compromised nutritional status in frail elderly patients. Clin Interv Aging 2006; 1(1):67–79.

64. Chiang JL, Kirkman MS, Laffel LM, et al, on behalf of the Type 1 Diabetes Sourcebook Authors. Type 1 diabetes through the life span: a position statement of the American Diabetes Association. Diabetes Care 2014;37(7):2034–54.

65. Pastors JG, Warshaw H, Daly A, et al. The evidence for the effectiveness of medical nutrition therapy in diabetes management. Diabetes Care 2002;25(3): 608–13.

66. Franz MJ, Boucher JL, Evert AB. Evidence-based diabetes nutrition therapy recommendations are effective: the key is individualization. Diabetes Metab Syndr Obes 2014;7:65–72.

67. Villareal DT, Apovian CM, Kushner RF, et al, American Society for Nutrition; NAASO, The Obesity Society. Obesity in older adults: technical review and position statement of the American Society for Nutrition and NAASO, The Obesity Society. Am J Clin Nutr 2005;82(5):923–34.

68. Suhl E, Bonsignore P. Diabetes self-management education for older adults: general principles and practical application. Diabetes Spectr 2006;19(4):234–40.

69. Scott R, O'Brien R, Fulcher G, et al. Fenofibrate Intervention and Event Lowering in Diabetes (FIELD) Study Investigators. Effects of fenofibrate treatment on cardiovascular disease risk in 9,795 individuals with type 2 diabetes and various components of the metabolic syndrome The Fenofibrate Intervention and Event Lowering in Diabetes (FIELD) study. Diabetes Care 2009;32(3):493–8.

70. Mann JF, Schmieder RE, McQueen M, et al. Renal outcomes with telmisartan, ramipril, or both, in people at high vascular risk (the ONTARGET study): a multicentre, randomised, double-blind, controlled trial. Lancet 2008;372(9638):547–53.

71. Mainous AG, Tanner RJ, Shorr RI, et al. Use of aspirin for primary and secondary cardiovascular disease prevention in the United States, 2011–2012. J Am Heart Assoc 2014;3(4). pii:e000989.

72. Smith SA, Poland GA, American Diabetes Association. Influenza and pneumo-coccal immunization in diabetes. Diabetes Care 2004;27(1):S111–3.
73. Centers for Disease Control and Prevention: Diabetes and Adult Vaccinations. 2014. Available at: http://www.cdc.gov/vaccines/hcp/patient-ed/adults/downloads/f-diabetes-vaccines.pdf. Accessed July 26, 2014.
74. Housden L, Wong ST, Dawes M. Effectiveness of group medical visits for improving diabetes care: a systematic review and meta-analysis. CMAJ 2013; 185(13):E635–44.
75. Suksomboon N, Poolsup N, Nge YL. Impact of phone call intervention on glyce-mic control in diabetes patients: a systematic review and meta-analysis of ran-domized, controlled trials. PLoS One 2014;9(2):e89207.
76. Health Quality Ontario. Home telemonitoring for type 2 diabetes: an evidence-based analysis. Ont Health Technol Assess Ser 2009;9(24):1–38.
77. Shea S, Weinstock RS, Teresi JA, et al, IDEATel Consortium. A randomized trial comparing telemedicine case management with usual care in older, ethnically diverse, medically underserved patients with diabetes mellitus: 5 year results of the IDEATel study. J Am Med Inform Assoc 2009;16(4):446–56.
78. Shea S, Kothari D, Teresi JA, et al. Social impact analysis of the effects of a tele-medicine intervention to improve diabetes outcomes in an ethnically diverse, medically underserved population: findings from the IDEATel Study. Am J Public Health 2013;103(10):1888–94.
79. Weinstock RS, Teresi JA, Goland R, et al, IDEATel Consortium. Glycemic control and health disparities in older ethnically diverse underserved adults with dia-betes: five-year results from the Informatics for Diabetes Education and Telemed-icine (IDEATel) study. Diabetes Care 2011;34(2):274–9.
80. Weinstock RS, Brooks G, Palmas W, et al. Lessened decline in physical activity and impairment of older adults with diabetes with telemedicine and pedometer use: results from the IDEATel study. Age Ageing 2011;40(1):98–105.
81. Luchsinger JA, Palmas W, Teresi JA, et al. Improved diabetes control in the elderly delays global cognitive decline. J Nutr Health Aging 2011;15(6):445–9.
82. Dy P, Morin PC, Weinstock RS. Use of telemedicine to improve glycemic manage-ment in a skilled nursing facility: a pilot study. Telemed J E Health 2013;19(8): 643–5.

Hypertension in the Geriatric Population
A Patient-Centered Approach

Philip A. Kithas, MD, PhD[a],*, Mark A. Supiano, MD[b]

KEYWORDS

• Hypertension • Elderly • Frailty • Guidelines • Goal blood pressure

KEY POINTS

• Goal blood pressure for healthy individuals age 60 to 80 years should be less than 140/90 mm Hg. Results of ongoing, randomized, controlled trials may modify this goal.

• Patients with multiple comorbidities, frailty, and/or diminished functional or cognitive status and those older than 80 years may be treated to a goal of less than 150/90 mm Hg.

• Lifestyle modifications should always be incorporated into antihypertensive therapy.

• The thiazide diuretic chlorthalidone should be the first-line agent for most older, hypertensive patients.

INTRODUCTION

The aging of the "baby boomer" population in conjunction with older individuals living longer means that the aging demographic imperative is a current reality. In 2011, the first of 77 million baby boomers turned 65 and approximately 10,000 Americans turn 65 on a daily basis. Three out of 4 adults older than the age of 65 have 3 or more chronic conditions such as diabetes (DM), obesity, cardiovascular disease, congestive heart failure, atrial fibrillation, stroke, cognitive impairment, renal insufficiency, and, not the least of which, hypertension. With the oldest old, those over 85 years of age, estimated to be the fastest growing part of the population over the next 40 years, the impact of hypertension and its consequences will be enormous.

When addressing the complexities of hypertension in older individuals, several considerations are apparent. When, or even if, treatment should be initiated and/or continued? What is the target blood pressure (BP) and should this be adjusted for

[a] George E. Wahlen Salt Lake Veterans Administration Medical Center, Geriatrics Division, University of Utah School of Medicine, 500 Foothill Drive, Salt Lake City, UT 84148, USA; [b] George E. Wahlen Department of Veterans Affairs Health Care System, VA Salt Lake City Geriatric Research, Education, and Clinical Center, Geriatrics Division, University of Utah School of Medicine, Salt Lake City GRECC (182), 500 Foothill Drive, Salt Lake City, UT 84148, USA
* Corresponding author.
E-mail address: Philip.Kithas@va.gov

Med Clin N Am 99 (2015) 379–389
http://dx.doi.org/10.1016/j.mcna.2014.11.009
0025-7125/15/$ – see front matter Published by Elsevier Inc.

medical.theclinics.com

comorbidities? Are benefits greater in those individuals who are less frail or have better functional status or gait speed than in those who do not? Does the risk of adverse outcomes ever outweigh the benefit? What is the role for nonpharmacologic interventions (exercise, a low-salt diet, and weight loss)? How much of a role does therapeutic inertia on the part of treating physicians play? Should time to benefit be taken into account, especially in those with a limited life expectancy or poor prognosis? Have obstructive sleep apnea and nocturnal hypertension been addressed as potential contributors? Finally, has a goals-of-care discussion taken place with the patient and his or her family in addressing these issues? To address these questions, along with what therapy is to be initiated and how aggressively, one must understand the various mechanisms contributing to hypertension in the older individual.

EPIDEMIOLOGY

Although not considered to be part of the normal aging process, there is a clear age-related increase in BP and in the prevalence of hypertension. According to the Framingham Heart Study,[1] in men and women with normal BP at age 55, 85% will develop hypertension over the next 20 to 25 years of follow-up. The results of the National Health and Nutrition Epidemiologic surveys also document the extremely high prevalence of hypertension among older Americans.[2] Based on their definition of hypertension—the average of 3 readings of 140 mm Hg systolic or greater and/or 90 mm Hg diastolic or greater or receiving antihypertensive medications—the overall prevalence of hypertension for those 65 years of age and older ranged from 50% to 75%. For women over age 75, the prevalence exceeded 75%.

PATHOPHYSIOLOGY

Hypertension in the geriatric population is typically characterized by a high systolic BP (SBP) in the setting of a normal or even decreased diastolic BP (**Fig. 1**). Both

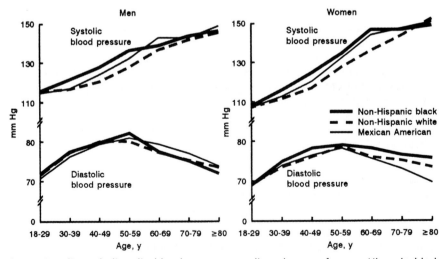

Fig. 1. Systolic and diastolic blood pressure readings by age for non-Hispanic black, non-Hispanic white, and Hispanic men and women from the Third National Health and Nutrition Evaluation Survey. (*From* Burt VL, Whelton P, Roccella EJ, et al. Prevalence of hypertension in the US adult population. Results from the Third National Health and Nutrition Examination Survey, 1988-1991. Hypertension 1995;25(3):305–13; with permission.)

elevated SBP and elevated pulse pressure (the difference between SBP and diastolic BP) are related to an age-related increase in arterial stiffness. No single factor accounts for this age-related increase in SBP. Although a detailed discussion is beyond the scope of this article, it is worth mentioning these factors, because several may serve as targets for both pharmacologic and nonpharmacologic interventions (**Box 1**). These vascular changes lead to an increase in central arterial stiffness demonstrated by higher arterial pulse wave velocity. Arterial stiffness in turn is believed to be a major contributor to target organ damage and impaired vascular function.

In addition to structural changes in the arteries, there are age-related changes in the autonomic nervous system along with impaired sensitivity of the arterial baroreceptors. As a consequence, a greater change in SBP is needed to elicit the appropriate compensatory response in heart rate and, for a given level of SBP, there is a more pronounced activation of the sympathetic nervous system. Reduced baroreceptor sensitivity has been proposed as a potential contributor to white coat hypertension, loss of the night time "dip" in BP,[3] greater BP variability and postprandial and orthostatic BP changes in the elderly.[4–6]

An age-related decline in renal function is well-documented and is accelerated in the setting of hypertension. A decline in renal cortical blood flow (~10% per decade) results in a loss of functioning glomeruli. Combined with an increase in pulse wave velocity, the remaining glomeruli are exposed to increased pressure transmitted through the small arterioles resulting in increased intraglomerular pressure and further loss of functional glomeruli. The decline in renal blood flow also leads to impaired ability to manage sodium loads. As a result, "salt sensitivity" ensues with an increase in mean arterial pressure of 5 mm Hg or more during a high compared with a low-salt diet.

With advancing age, there are also changes in the renin–angiotensin–aldosterone system associated with increased BP and salt sensitivity. Until end-stage renal disease develops, hypertension in the elderly is characterized by low renin activity. The effects of aldosterone are likely multifactorial (eg, vascular stiffness, central obesity, impaired endothelial function), but increasing levels within the physiologic range may predict the development of hypertension in normotensive subjects.

Box 1
Factors in the age-related increase in blood pressure

Arterial stiffness: Hypertrophy and loss of contractility of vascular smooth muscle cells, fibrosis, collagen deposition, fragmentation of elastic lamina, calcification

Decreased baroreceptor sensitivity

Increased sympathetic nervous system activity

Increased α-adrenergic receptor responsiveness

Endothelial dysfunction: Decreased nitric oxide production

Sodium sensitivity: Decreased ability to excrete a sodium load

Low plasma renin activity

Insulin resistance

Central adiposity

Adapted from Halter J, Ouslander J, Tinetti M, et al, editors. Hazzard's Geriatric Medicine and Gerontology. 6th edition. New York: McGraw-Hill; 2009.

DIAGNOSTIC CONSIDERATIONS

To ensure that appropriate treatment decisions are made, it is imperative that accurate BP measurement take place. Guidelines for accurate BP measurement not only specify appropriate cuff size and type of instrument, but emphasize the need for repeated measurements before making the diagnosis.[7] Indeed, the greater variability of BP in the elderly dictates that the diagnosis of hypertension should be based on the average of at least 3 readings (with the first discarded and subsequent readings averaged) at 3 separate visits over a period of 4 to 6 weeks (provided the presenting BP is not 180/110 mm Hg or greater).

The presence of an auscultatory gap, which is strongly associated with arterial stiffness, may lead to a significant underestimation of the true SBP. The gap represents a temporary loss of Korotkoff sounds between phase 2 and 3 and may span anywhere from a few to greater than 20 mm Hg. The auscultatory gap can be detected by palpating either the radial or brachial artery during rapid manual cuff inflation to a pressure 30 mm Hg above the value where the pulse is no longer palpable. Then, during auscultation for Korotkoff sounds, the cuff is deflated slowly at 1 to 2 mm Hg per second. Determination of BP by using electronic oscillometric devices is not affected by the auscultatory gap because they measure mean arterial pressure, which in turn is used to calculate an estimate of SBP and DBP.[8]

Orthostatic or postural hypotension (a drop in SBP or DBP of $\geq$20 mm Hg or 10 mm Hg, respectively, within 2–3 minutes of standing) was present in 8% of the participants in the Hypertension in the Very Elderly Trial (HYVET),[9] but may be even more prevalent in unselected patients with hypertension.[10] For this reason, supine, sitting, and upright BP should always be obtained and incorporated into treatment decisions because the presence of systolic orthostasis in older individuals with uncontrolled hypertension predicts an increased risk for falls within 1 year.[11]

With the prevalence of office or white coat hypertension in the community reaching 20% to 25%, it is imperative that an accurate diagnosis be reached. This diagnosis applies specifically to untreated individuals with office BPs of 140/90 mm Hg or higher but who have 24-hour ambulatory BP of less than 130/80 mm Hg (awake <135/85 mm Hg, sleep <120/70 mm Hg) or home BP of less than 135/85 mm Hg.[12] Therefore, further evaluation by way of careful home BP or 24-hour ambulatory BP monitoring is indicated in this population. Twenty-four hour BP monitoring not only provides the overall average BP, but has the added advantage of defining daytime and nocturnal averages. Although the 24-hour average correlates with indicators of target organ damage and BP load, the lack of at least a 10% drop in the nocturnal relative to the daytime average BP (nondippers) predicts a greater cardiovascular disease risk compared with the normal dipping pattern.

BLOOD PRESSURE CONTROL AND OUTCOMES

The Prospective Studies Collaboration, a meta-analysis of 61 prospective observational studies evaluating vascular mortality in subjects without vascular disease at baseline, demonstrated a positive association of SBP and DBP with stroke and ischemic heart disease over 4 decades of age from 50 to 59 to 80 to 89. A 20-mm Hg increase in SBP was associated with a 10-fold greater annual absolute stroke risk in patients in their 80s compared with those in their 50s (**Fig. 2**).[13] Based on their findings, the authors state that "blood-pressure-lowering treatment should be considered for a wide range of patients with evidence of occlusive vascular disease, largely irrespective of their current BP or the use of other medication." Given the increasing incidence of cardiovascular disease in the elderly population, one must consider

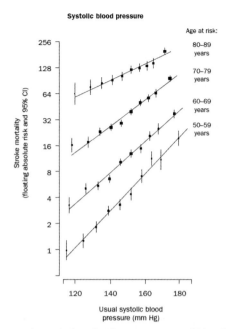

Systolic blood pressure

Fig. 2. Stroke mortality rate in each decade of age versus usual blood pressure at the start of that decade. (*From* Lewington S, Clarke R, Qizilbash N, et al. Age-specific relevance of usual blood pressure to vascular mortality: a meta-analysis of individual data for one million adults in 61 prospective studies. Lancet 2002;360(9349):1906; with permission.)

that even a modest reduction in relative risk with treating hypertension may lead to a considerable decrease in absolute risk. Multiple hypertension trials in the older populations have supported this conclusion.[9,14–20]

The landmark HYVET demonstrated that antihypertensive therapy in patients over the age of 80 years led to improved outcomes in stroke, cardiovascular events, heart failure, and death with a goal BP of less than 150/80 mm Hg. The HYVET population had fewer comorbid illnesses and was generally healthier than average, such that its results may not generalize to the significant number of older patients with poor functional status, frailty, multiple medical problems, and cognitive impairment/dementia who do not meet inclusion criteria for most randomized, controlled trials. What BP goals should be used in this heterogeneous population and can we identify those who will benefit from achieving lower values through treatment versus those better off left untreated? Although the positive association of high BP and increased cardiovascular risk is maintained into older age, it may diminish or even reverse in those older individuals with poor functional status or those who are frail.

Prospective, population-based cohort studies have found conflicting results, particularly in the oldest old (those ≥85 years), and demonstrate an inverse association between hypertension and mortality in higher age groups. In the Leiden 85-plus study, a low SBP (≤150 mm Hg) predicted increased mortality in a 90-year-old population, regardless of their N-terminal prohormone of brain natriuretic peptide level.[21] A consistent finding in several studies was an attenuation or even reversal of the association of hypertension and cardiovascular risk in the age range of 75 to 85 years.[22–25]

What might explain the differences in these studies? A potential explanation lies in the differences between study populations. The prospective cohort studies mentioned included individuals with multiple medical problems, dependency in activities of daily living and instrumental activities of daily living, and cognitive and functional impairment, as well as some who were institutionalized, all of which contribute to frailty. By comparison, the Prospective Studies Collaboration included subjects with a higher overall general health status and lesser prevalence of comorbid illnesses.

Gait speed, as a surrogate for frailty in 2340 individuals age 65 and older, was used to predict which subjects might be at greater risk for the adverse effects of hypertension and who subsequently may benefit from intervention.[26] Among those with a faster gait speed (≥0.8 m/s) a SBP of 140 mm Hg or greater was associated with an increased risk for mortality. Among slower walkers, no association between elevated SBP or DBP and mortality was observed. Interestingly, for those who could not complete the walk test an elevated SBP and DBP was independently associated with a lower mortality risk.

Among 4961 community-dwelling adults older than 70 years (mean age, 80) with hypertension and multiple medical comorbidities, use of antihypertensive medication was associated with an increase in serious fall injuries (hip and other major fractures, traumatic brain injuries, joint dislocations). Compared with no medication, the administration of moderate to high doses of any anti-hypertensive was associated with a 30% to 40% increased risk of falls with injury. This association was even stronger among those with a history of previous fall injury.[27]

WHAT DO CURRENT GUIDELINES RECOMMEND?

The Joint National Committee on Prevention, Detection, Evaluation and Treatment of High Blood Pressure (JNC 7)[28] was published in 2003 and, in the general population without DM or chronic kidney disease (CKD) recommended the same goal BP of less than 140/90 mm Hg in patients older than 65 years as for younger patients. In 2013, 4 other organizations, including the American Society of Hypertension and International society of Hypertension,[29] European Society of Hypertension and European Society of Cardiology,[30] Canadian Hypertension Education Program,[31] and the American Diabetes Association[32] published their guidelines, each of which promulgates the same less than 140/90 mm Hg target goal (**Table 1**).[33] The 2014 Evidence-Based Guideline for the Management of High Blood Pressure in Adults:

Table 1
Summary of major hypertension guidelines: Goal blood pressure (mm Hg)

Age (y)	JNC-7[28] (2003)	ASH/ISH[29] (2013)	ESH/ESC[30] (2013)	CHEP[31] (2013)	JNC-8[34] (2014)
<60 y	<140/90	<140/90	<140/90	<140/90	<140/90
60–79	<140/90	<140/90	<140/90	<140/90	<150/90
≥80	<140/90	<150/90	<150/90	<150/90	<150/90

These guidelines apply to patients without chronic kidney disease or diabetes.
Abbreviations: ASH/ISH, American Society of Hypertension and International society of Hypertension; CHEP, Canadian Hypertension Education Program; ESH/ESC, European Society of Hypertension and European Society of Cardiology; JNC-7, Joint National Committee on Prevention, Detection, Evaluation and Treatment of High Blood Pressure.
Adapted from Salvo M, White CM. Reconciling multiple hypertension guidelines to promote effective clinical practice. Ann Pharmacotherapy 2014;48:1243.

Report From the Panel Members Appointed to the Eighth Joint National Committee (also known as JNC-8)[34] recommended a goal BP of less than 150/90 mm Hg in patients without DM or CKD between the ages of 60 and 80 years. However, significant controversy surrounds the most recent guidelines and their recommendations not only in the population age 60 to 79 without DM or CKD, but also in women and African Americans.

With regard to raising the goal SBP from 140 to 150 mm Hg in the population between 60 and 80 years of age without DM or CKD, 5 members of the JNC-8 panel published a dissenting opinion.[35] In arguing for a continued goal of less than 140 mm Hg, several points were made. First, an increase in the target SBP to 150 mm Hg in a population at high risk for cardiovascular disease might lead to a reduction in the intensity of anti-hypertensive therapy. Coronary heart disease (CHD) risk increases with age and SBP has a much more significant impact on CHD risk than total cholesterol at older ages. Therefore, a different target BP in individuals age 60 and over compared with those younger than 60 is not justified. In addition, evidence supporting the increased SBP goal in this population was felt to be "insufficient and inconsistent" with that supporting the recommendation for a goal of less than 140 mm Hg in those younger than 60 or over age 60 with DM or CKD. Second, the decline in cardiovascular disease, especially stroke mortality, seen over the last several years might be reversed by a higher SBP goal. Third, the current guidelines are not in keeping with goals put forth in the guidelines from the majority of organizations listed herein.

In African Americans, a population with increased prevalence of CHD, stroke, CKD, and heart failure, the relaxation of the SBP goal to less than 150 mm Hg would likely result in an increase in major adverse cardiovascular outcomes and end-organ damage, especially in elderly blacks and is opposed by the Association of Black Cardiologists. Of note, the 2010 International Society of Hypertension in Blacks consensus statement recommends instituting therapy at BP level of greater than 135/85 mm Hg.[36]

Among patients over age 60 with hypertension in the United States, women represent the majority. Within this population, hypertension is the most significant contributor to heart failure, stroke, DM, CKD, and CHD. Raising the SBP goal to less than 150 mm Hg in women, African Americans, and the healthy older population would negatively impact cardiovascular outcomes and place these populations at unnecessary excess risk.[37]

THERAPY: NONPHARMACOLOGIC TREATMENT OPTIONS

Lifestyle modifications, including weight loss, physical exercise, and a low-salt diet, should be recommended to all patients with hypertension. The Trial of Nonpharmacologic Intervention in the Elderly (TONE)[38] demonstrated that modest reductions in sodium intake (average of 40 mmol/d) and weight loss (average 4 kg) lead to a 30% decrease in the need to reinitiate antihypertensive medication in the intervention group. A reduction in dietary sodium based on the Dietary Approaches to Stop Hypertension (DASH) diet has been shown to reduce BP in untreated hypertensives,[39] prehypertensives,[40] and in older patients with heart failure with preserved ejection fraction.[41] Lifestyle modifications will be adjunctive to pharmacotherapy, lead to improvement in other cardiovascular risk factors such as hyperlipidemia, and may improve physical and cognitive function. Weight loss, aerobic exercise, and reductions in salt and alcohol intake have all demonstrated sustained benefit in BP reduction and each averages a 5 mm Hg reduction in SBP, which is comparable with intervention with a single antihypertensive agent.

PHARMACOLOGIC TREATMENT OPTIONS

In considering the treatment of hypertension in older patients, multiple issues must be taken into account. As discussed, there seems to be a difference in cardiovascular risk and benefit from therapy between those older individuals with preserved functional status and those with impaired function or frailty. In addition, there are concerns related to polypharmacy, potential drug–drug interactions, cognitive impairment, and increasing medical comorbidities. Also, the presence of orthostatic hypotension and sleep apnea need to be taken into consideration. The willingness of the patient and/or their family to monitor home BP values must also be taken into account. Because the benefit of BP lowering is seen within the first year of therapy, a goals-of-care discussion in those with limited life expectancy or on hospice care is imperative.

Given these considerations and current data, we favor the approach to initiating therapy recommended by the EHS/ESC and Canadian Hypertension Education Program (see **Table 1**). The first-line therapeutic class that is recommended by the majority of guidelines in patients over age 60, without compelling medical indications such as DM and coronary artery disease, is a thiazide diuretic. Within this category the preferred agent would be chlorthalidone over hydrochlorothiazide owing to its greater potency and longer half-life, as well as evidence of greater efficacy from multiple randomized, controlled trials.[42] Additional, or second-line agents, would include angiotensin converting enzyme inhibitors, angiotensin receptor blockers, and both dihydropyridine and nondihydropyridine calcium channel blockers. β-Blockers are clearly indicated in those older individuals with underlying coronary artery disease and/or congestive heart failure, but are otherwise not indicated as first-line agents. Recommended approaches to treating the oldest old based on the currently available data have also been proposed with the caveat that they represent subjective views and are not based on firm evidence provided by randomized, controlled trials.[43]

SUMMARY

The approach to hypertension in the geriatric population should be no different than that of other geriatric syndromes. Hypertension in older people represents a heterogeneous physiologic process and should be approached on an individual, case-by-case basis. Given the current level of uncertainty regarding the appropriate SBP goal in the hypertensive patient over age 60 without DM or CKD, data are needed from large, randomized, controlled trials. The ongoing SPRINT (Systolic Blood Pressure Intervention Trial) and ESH-CHL-SHOT (Optimal Blood Pressure and Cholesterol Targets for Preventing Recurrent Stroke in Hypertensives) are two such studies. Both trials will compare a goal SBP of near 140 mm Hg with lower SBP goals. While awaiting these results, we recommend a goal SBP of less than 140 mm Hg in the healthy hypertensive population between the ages of 60 and 80 years and emphasize that risk–benefit considerations be incorporated into decision making in those with poor physical or cognitive function and/or frailty.

REFERENCES

1. Vasan RS, Beiser A, Seshadri S, et al. Residual lifetime risk for developing hypertension in middle-aged men and women: the Framingham heart study. JAMA 2002;287:1003–10.

2. Ostchega Y, Dillon CF, Hughes JP, et al. Trends in hypertension prevalence, awareness, treatment, and control in older U.S. adults: data from the National Health and Nutrition Examination Survey 1988 to 2004. J Am Geriatr Soc 2007; 55:1056–65.
3. Franklin SS. Elderly hypertensives: how are they different? J Clin Hypertens (Greenwich) 2012;14:779–86.
4. James MA, Potter JF. Orthostatic blood pressure changes and arterial baroreflex sensitivity in elderly subjects. Age Ageing 1999;28:522–30.
5. Bertinieri G, Grassi G, Rossi P, et al. 24-hour blood pressure profile in centenarians. J Hypertens 2002;20:1765–9.
6. Vloet LC, Pel-Little RE, Jansen PA, et al. High prevalence of post-prandial and orthostatic hypotension among geriatric patients admitted to Dutch hospitals. J Gerontol A Biol Sci Med Sci 2005;60:1271–7.
7. Dasgupta K, Quinn RR, Zarnke KT, et al. The 2014 Canadian hypertension education program recommendations for blood pressure measurement, diagnosis, assessment of risk prevention, and treatment of hypertension. Can J Cardiol 2014;30:485–501.
8. Frech TM, Penrod J, Battistone MJ, et al. The prevalence and clinical correlates of an auscultatory gap in systemic sclerosis patients. Int J Rheum Dis 2012; 2012:1–4.
9. Beckett NS, Peters R, Fletcher AE, et al, HYVET Study Group. Treatment of hypertension in patients 80 years of age or older. N Engl J Med 2008;358:1887–98.
10. Feldstein C, Weder AB. Orthostatic hypotension: a common, serious and underrecognized problem in hospitalized patients. J Am Soc Hypertens 2012;6:27–39.
11. Gangavati A, Hajjar I, Quach L, et al. Hypertension, orthostatic hypotension, and the risk of falls in a community-dwelling elderly population: the maintenance of balance, independent living, intellect, and zest in the Elderly of Boston Study. J Am Geriatr Soc 2011;59:383–9.
12. Parati G, Stergiou G, O'Brien E, et al. European society of hypertension practice guidelines for ambulatory blood pressure monitoring. J Hypertens 2014;32: 1359–66.
13. Lewington S, Clarke R, Qizilbash N, et al, Prospective Studies Collaboration. Age-specific relevance of usual blood pressure to vascular mortality; a meta-analysis of individual data for one million adults in 61 prospective studies. Lancet 2002; 360:1903–13.
14. Amery A, Birkenhager W, Brixko P, et al. Mortality and morbidity results from the European Working Party on High Blood Pressure in the Elderly trial. Lancet 1985; 1:1349–54.
15. Prevention of stroke by antihypertensive drug treatment in older persons with isolated systolic hypertension. Final results of the Systolic Hypertension in the Elderly Program (SHEP). SHEP Cooperative Research Group. JAMA 1991;265: 3255–64.
16. Dahlof B, Lindholm LH, Hansson L, et al. Morbidity and mortality in the Swedish Trial in Old Patients with Hypertension (STOP-Hypertension). Lancet 1991;338:1281–5.
17. Staessen JA, Fagard R, Thijs L, et al. Randomised double-blind comparison of placebo and active treatment for older patients with isolated systolic hypertension. The systolic Hypertension in Europe (Syst-Eur) Trial Investigators. Lancet 1997;350:757–64.
18. Liu L, Wang JG, Gong L, et al. Comparison of active treatment and placebo in older Chinese patients with isolated systolic hypertension. Systolic Hypertension in China (Syst-China) Collaborative Group. J Hypertens 1998;16:1823–9.

19. Medical Research Council trial of treatment of hypertension in older adults; principle results. MRC Working Party. BMJ 1992;304:405–12.

20. Ogihara T, Saruta T, Rakugi H, et al, Valsartan in Elderly Isolated Systolic Hypertension Study Group. Target blood pressure for treatment of isolated systolic hypertension in the elderly: valsartan in elderly isolated systolic hypertension study. Hypertension 2010;56:196–202.

21. Poortvliet RK, Blom JW, de Craen AJ, et al. Low blood pressure predicts increased mortality in very old age even without heart failure: the Leiden 85-plus Study. Eur J Heart Fail 2013;15:528–33.

22. van Bemmel T, Gussekloo J, Westendorp RG, et al. In a population-based prospective study, no association between high blood pressure and mortality after age 85 years. J Hypertens 2006;24:287–92.

23. Poortvliet RK, de Ruijter W, de Craen AJ, et al. Blood pressure trends and mortality: the Leiden 85-plus Study. J Hypertens 2013;31:63–70.

24. Satish S, Freeman DH, Ray L, et al. The relationship between blood pressure and mortality in the oldest old. J Am Geriatr Soc 2001;49:367–74.

25. Mattila K, Haavisto M, Rajala S, et al. Blood pressure and five year survival in the very old. BMJ 1988;296:887–9.

26. Odden MC, Peralta CA, Haan MN, et al. Rethinking the association of high blood pressure with mortality in elderly adults. The impact of frailty. Arch Intern Med 2012;172:1162–8.

27. Tinetti ME, Han L, Lee DS, et al. Antihypertensive medications and serious fall injuries in a nationally representative sample of older adults. JAMA Intern Med 2014;174:588–95.

28. Chobanian AV, Bakris G, Black HR, et al. The seventh report of the Joint National Committee on Prevention, Detection, Evaluation, and Treatment of High Blood Pressure. JAMA 2003;289:2560–72.

29. Weber MA, Schiffrin EL, White WB, et al. Clinical practice guidelines for the management of hypertension in the community: a statement by the American Society of Hypertension and the International society of Hypertension. J Clin Hypertens (Greenwich) 2014;16:14–26.

30. Mancia G, Fagard R, Narkiewicz K, et al. 2013 ESH/ESC guidelines for the management of arterial hypertension. Eur Heart J 2013;34:2159–219.

31. Hypertension without compelling indications: 2013 CHEP Recommendations. Hypertension Canada Website. Available at: https://www.hypertension.ca/en/professional/chep/therapy/hypertension-without-compelling-indications. Accessed December 15, 2014.

32. American Diabetes Association. Standards of medical care in diabetes-2013. Diabetes Care 2013;35(Suppl 1):s11–66.

33. Salvo M, White CM. Reconciling multiple hypertension guidelines to promote effective clinical practice. Ann Pharmacother 2014;48:1242–8.

34. James PA, Oparil S, Carter B, et al. 2014 Evidence-based guideline for the management of high blood pressure in adults: Report from the Panel Members Appointed to the Eighth Joint National Committee (JNC 8). JAMA 2014;311:507–20.

35. Wrigth JT, Fin LJ, Lackland DT, et al. Evidence supporting a systolic blood pressure goal of less than 150 mm Hg in patients aged 60 years or older: the minority view. Ann Intern Med 2014;160:499–503.

36. Flack JM, Sica DA, Bakris G, et al. Management of high blood pressure in African Americans: management of high blood pressure in blacks: an update of the International Society on Hypertension in Blacks Consensus Statement. Hypertension 2010;56:780–800.

37. Krakoff LF, Gillespie RL, Ferdinand KC, et al. 2014 hypertension recommendations from the Eighth Joint National Committee Panel Members raise concerns for elderly black and female populations. J Am Coll Cardiol 2014;64:394–402.
38. Whelton PK, Appel LJ, Espeland MA, et al. Sodium reduction and weight loss in the treatment of hypertension in older persons: a randomized controlled trial of nonpharmacologic interventions in the elderly (TONE). JAMA 1998;279:839–46.
39. Sacks FM, Svetkey LP, Vollmer WM, et al. Effects on blood pressure of reduced dietary sodium and the Dietary Approaches to Stop Hypertension (DASH) diet. N Engl J Med 2001;344:3–10.
40. Al-Solaiman Y, Jesri A, Shao Y, et al. Low-Sodium DASH reduces oxidative stress and improves vascular function in salt-sensitive humans. J Hum Hypertens 2009; 23:826–35.
41. Hummel SL, Seymour EM, Brook RD, et al. Low-sodium dietary approaches to stop hypertension diet reduces blood pressure, arterial stiffness, and oxidative stress in hypertensive heart failure with preserved ejection fraction. Hypertension 2012;60:1200–6.
42. Roush GC, Holford TR, Guddati AK. Chlorthalidone compared with hydrochlorothiazide in reducing cardiovascular events: systematic review and network meta-analyses. Hypertension 2012;59(6):1110–7.
43. Muller M, Smulders YM, de Leeuw PW, et al. Treatment of hypertension in the oldest old. A critical role for frailty? Hypertension 2014;64:1–9.

Advance Care Planning in the Elderly

Hillary D. Lum, MD, PhD[a,b,*], Rebecca L. Sudore, MD[c], David B. Bekelman, MD, MPH[d,e]

KEYWORDS

- Advance care planning • Advance directives • Surrogate decision maker
- Patient-doctor relationship • Communication

KEY POINTS

- Advance care planning (ACP) can help individuals and their loved ones receive medical care that is aligned with their values, and experience more satisfaction and peace of mind.
- ACP involves a process identifying personal values first, and then translating those values into medical care plans.
- ACP can be viewed as a health behavior that involves multiple steps and evolves as a process over time.
- Clinicians can assist older adults with ACP through assessing readiness, promoting identification and documentation of appropriate surrogate decision makers, engaging patients and surrogates in discussions, and helping patients document their medical wishes.
- Outpatient approaches to support ACP can be brief, multidisciplinary, and involve several visits over time.

INTRODUCTION

Advance care planning (ACP) allows individuals to specify in advance how they want to be treated should serious illness prevent them from being able to make decisions or communicate their choices. Just as tobacco cessation counseling could be considered a primary care provider's "procedure," engaging patients and their potential surrogate decision makers in ACP is a key skill in the care of the older adult. ACP involves multiple conversations that identify a surrogate decision maker, explore the individual's values about medical care, complete advance directive documents, and

[a] Division of Geriatric Medicine, Department of Medicine, University of Colorado School of Medicine, 12631 East 17th Avenue, B-179, Aurora, CO 80045, USA; [b] Department of Medicine, VA Eastern Colorado Healthcare System, 1055 Clermont Street, Denver, CO 80220, USA; [c] Division of Geriatrics, San Francisco VA Medical Center, University of California, 4150 Clement Street, #151R, San Francisco, CA 94121, USA; [d] Department of Medicine, Division of General Internal Medicine, University of Colorado School of Medicine, 12631 East 17th Avenue, Aurora, CO 80045, USA; [e] Department of Medicine, VA Eastern Colorado Healthcare System, 1055 Clermont Street, Research (151), Denver, CO 80220, USA
* Corresponding author. 12631 East 17th Avenue, B-179, Aurora, CO 80045.
E-mail address: Hillary.Lum@ucdenver.edu

Med Clin N Am 99 (2015) 391–403
http://dx.doi.org/10.1016/j.mcna.2014.11.010
0025-7125/15/$ – see front matter Published by Elsevier Inc.

medical.theclinics.com

translate values into medical care plans. This article describes the need for ACP in the elderly and highlights several key concepts for clinicians to assist older adults with ACP. Practical approaches for integrating ACP into busy primary care practices are provided, while recognizing common barriers, and recently developed ACP tools for clinicians and the outpatient care team are highlighted.

WHAT IS ADVANCE CARE PLANNING?

ACP is the process of planning for future medical care with the goal of helping patients receive medical care that is aligned with their preferences, especially in the setting of serious illness or as the end of life approaches. **Table 1** provides common terms and definitions used in ACP. For example, one component of ACP is advance directives, which include medical power of attorney appointments or living wills; these written forms facilitate end-of-life decision making based on a patient's values. Fundamentally ACP involves more than completing an advance directive in isolation because ACP is based on an individual's evolving values regarding future medical care, not only their preference for particular medical procedures, such as cardiopulmonary

Table 1 Advance care planning terms and definitions	
Advance Care Planning Terms	**Description of Terms**
Advance care planning (ACP)	Process of considering and communicating health care values and goals over time
Advance directive	Legal document describing preferences for future care and appointing a surrogate to make health care decisions in the event of incapacity
Medical durable power of attorney	Legal documents that appoints an "agent" to make future medical decisions. Becomes effective only when the patient becomes incapacitated
Surrogate decision maker or health care proxy	A decision maker that makes medical decisions when the patient becomes incapacitated and the individual did not previously identify a medical durable power of attorney. Most states use a hierarchy system to designate a health care proxy, whereas a few states appoint a proxy that is agreed on by all interested parties
Living will	Documents an individual's wishes prospectively regarding initiating, withholding, and withdrawing certain life-sustaining medical interventions. Effective when the patient becomes incapacitated and has certain medical conditions
Cardiopulmonary resuscitation (CPR) directive or do-not-resuscitate (DNR) order	Documents preferences to refuse unwanted resuscitation attempts
Orders for life-sustaining treatment (ie, Physicians Orders for Life-Sustaining Treatment [POLST] paradigm)	Order set that translates patient preferences for life-sustaining therapies into medical orders Primarily intended for seriously ill people with life-limiting or terminal illnesses and patients in long-term care facilities Portable and transferable between health care settings

resuscitation (CPR), in specific settings and at one point in time. Thus, the process of ACP involves conversations with family, friends, and clinicians over time, and is much more than a one-time documentation of advance directives. Although the benefits of advance directives in isolation remain controversial,[1,2] recent evidence suggests that ACP conversations and support achieve a range of benefits, including fulfillment of end-of-life wishes and higher patient and family satisfaction.[3–5] Key concepts of the ACP process are summarized in **Table 2** and are discussed later in this article.

THE NEED FOR ADVANCE CARE PLANNING IN THE ELDERLY

Benefits of ACP include the following:

- Ability to identify, respect, and implement an individual's wishes for medical care, especially in the absence of decision-making capacity, during serious illness, or near the end of life[2]
- Ability to manage personal affairs while able, peace of mind, less burden on loved ones, and peace within the family[6]
- Reduction in stress, anxiety, and depression in surviving family members[4]
- Improved patient satisfaction and quality of life[7,8]
- Decreased use of intensive medical interventions at the end of life[7,8]
- Implementation of preferences to limit unwanted medical treatment (eg, avoid hospitalization or CPR)[9]
- Fewer in-hospital deaths, more hospice use, and lower Medicare costs among older adults, with advance directives specifying comfort-oriented end-of-life care[5,10,11]

A growing evidence base supports the benefits of specific systematic approaches to ACP. For example, Respecting Choices, a trained facilitator-based model whereby individuals engage in multiple ACP conversations, has been successfully implemented into a health care system and has increased the prevalence of advance directives to 90% in the local community.[3,12,13] Respecting Choices has also improved the delivery of goal-concordant end-of-life care through an emphasis on conversations that go far beyond completing advance directives. Another major success related to ACP has been implementation of out-of-hospital orders for medical treatment, such as Physicians Orders for Life-Sustaining Treatment (POLST) forms, which necessitate a doctor-patient discussion about individual preferences for medical care.[9,14,15]

Despite the proven benefits of ACP, many older adults with chronic illnesses die after extended periods of disability, without prior ACP with their family or primary care provider. In 1995, 20% of hospitalized patients had an advance directive, and of those with an advance directive only 12% had been counseled by a physician about writing the directive.[16] Many physicians and surrogate decision makers were unaware of patients' preferences.[17] Although the percentage of older adults completing advance directives has increased over time, there is still a poor correlation between wishes expressed in these documents, documentation in the medical record, and the care individuals receive at the end of life. For example, in recent national studies as many as 70% of elderly decedents had an advance directive,[18] although the presence of an advance directive had little effect on hospitalization rates within 2 years of death.[19] Although the number of deaths in United States hospitals has declined, this trend was not associated with the increased completion of advance directives after adjusting for sociodemographic characteristics. Among hospitalized patients in Canada, concordance between patients' expressed preferences for end-of-life care and documentation in the medical record was only 30.2%.[20] This poor correlation between

Table 2
Advance care planning is a multistep process

Key Concept	Description	Examples of Questions to Engage Patients in ACP Discussions
Assessing readiness and identifying barriers	Exploring patient readiness and identifying and addressing any barriers to the ACP process	"Have you ever completed an advance directive, like a living will? What did it say? Is it up-to-date?" "ACP helps me work with you and your family to understand how to plan your medical care in case you lose the ability to make decisions. Can we talk about this today?" "Are there things that you worry about when you think about planning for future medical care?[26] What keeps you from thinking about these types of things?"
Identifying surrogate decision makers	Identifying a trusted person as a surrogate decision maker to help clinicians apply overarching care goals to specific clinical situations in the event that the patient loses decisional capacity.	"Is there someone you trust to be involved in making medical decisions on your behalf, if you are not able to do so?" "What have you talked about?" or "What would you tell this person is important about your medical care?" "Flexibility gives your decision maker leeway to work with your doctors and possibly change your prior medical decisions if something else is better for you at that time. Are there decisions about your health that you would not want your loved one to change?"
Asking about patient's values related to quality of life	Exploring the individual's values and priorities in life, and discussing what constitutes an acceptable quality of life	"Have you had any previous experience with making decisions about medical care during a serious illness? Can you tell me about that?" "When (eg, you were hospitalized; loved one died), did this situation change your thoughts about what is important to you in the future or what would be unacceptable, where you wouldn't want to live like that?"

(continued on next page)

| | | Examples of Questions to Engage Patients in ACP |
Key Concept	Description	Discussions
Documenting ACP preferences	Documenting expressed care preferences in an advance directive document (eg, medical power of attorney, living will); ensuring written plans are communicated, stored, and retrievable	"Since you've chosen (loved one) to help make decisions on your behalf if you're very sick and unable to talk with me, I recommend that you complete the medical power of attorney form to make it official." "Can you bring in your advance directives? It helps me, the clinic, and the hospital, know what is important to you if you are very sick."
Translating preferences into medical care plans	Translating values and preferences into current medical care documents (ie, POLST form, CPR directive); documenting discussions, preferences, and care plans in the medical record	"You told me that if you were not able to interact with your family and friends, your life would not be worth living. Did I get that right? Many patients who feel as you do, opt not to have life support treatments if they become so sick they cannot recognize family. Based on what you told about what is important to you, I'd like to go through the POLST form if that's OK so that (emergency medical services, other doctors) know what you want." "At this point, (medical intervention) is no longer providing you with benefit. Given what you have told me, I recommend that we focus on treatments that maximize your quality of life (such as…) and stop (medical intervention)."

Table 2
(continued)

Adapted from Refs.[25,26,28,43,50]

advance directive completion, medical record documentation of preferences, and care provided at the end of life support the need for novel, practical, and systematic approaches for integrating ACP into health care systems.

Clinician and Health Care System Barriers to Advance Care Planning

Despite the benefits of ACP, clinicians face significant barriers to engaging patients in ACP. Personalized, comprehensive ACP involves conversations between clinicians and patient or surrogate decision makers that can be time consuming. In one study, primary care providers described barriers such as variation in how providers approach

ACP, lack of useful information about patient values to guide decision making, and ineffective communication between providers across settings.[21] Although patients infrequently initiate these discussions, clinicians missed opportunities to engage in ACP discussions when patients expressed concerns regarding their future care.[22] Health care systems often lack the personnel or work flow processes to systematically approach ACP. The Affordable Care Act instituted a requirement for ACP during Medicare Annual Wellness visits, but there are no evidence-based guidelines to direct this process or consensus on appropriate patient-centered outcomes. Furthermore, the lack of specific reimbursement for ACP counseling, especially if completed by ancillary staff, is a significant limitation in clinical practice.

Nonetheless, older adults with chronic illnesses described the importance of preparing for medical decision making and were more satisfied with their primary care physicians when ACP was discussed.[7,23] Primary care settings remain a critical opportunity to engage older patients and surrogate decision makers in ACP discussions.[24] Older adults experience significant life, social, and health-related changes that may lead to increased awareness of the need and readiness for ACP. **Box 1** highlights opportunities to initiate or revisit ACP in older adult patients.

KEY CONCEPTS IN ADVANCE CARE PLANNING

Key steps in ACP are (1) assessing patient readiness and identifying barriers, (2) identifying surrogate decision makers, (3) asking about individuals' values related to quality of life and serious illness, (4) documenting ACP preferences, and (5) translating individuals' preferences into medical care plans. **Table 2** summarizes brief approaches to each key concept.

ACP is a stepwise process that does not need to occur in a single clinic visit; it is a process that can unfold over time. For instance, clinicians and outpatient staff can engage older adults in ACP through introducing key concepts over time. Each concept can be discussed individually and in 5 minutes, based on time constraints and patient needs, and can be used by trained staff members as part of team-based or health care system–based approaches (see later discussion).

Assessing Patient Readiness and Identifying Barriers

Engaging an individual in ACP can begin with assessing patient readiness. Studies show that patients are in varying stages of readiness to engage in ACP,[6,25,26] and often barriers may need to be addressed before patients can engage. **Table 2** suggests

---

Box 1
Indications for advance care planning (ACP) in the elderly patient

- Medicare Annual Wellness examination (ie, routine preventive visits)
- Diagnosis of mild cognitive impairment or early dementia
- Need for increased caregiver involvement
- Identification of new functional impairment
- Transition to an assisted living facility or nursing home
- Post-hospitalization, post–subacute rehabilitation, or other care transition
- Change (decline or improvement) in health status
- Changes in family or social situation, including death of loved ones

brief opening questions that explore the patient's readiness through understanding their past experiences with ACP. The process can be introduced alongside other common future planning considerations (ie, financial planning, place of residence). Questions should be tailored to the individual's clinical context, such as new medical diagnoses, increased care needs, or changes in social support. Responses of patients or available family members can help clinicians identify how ready patients are to engage in the ACP process (**Table 3**), and lead clinicians to appropriate next ACP steps or, if the patient is not ready, asking permission to revisit in the future.

Table 2 provides examples of open-ended questions to help identify barriers. There are many reasons why patients and families may be reluctant to address difficult or frightening health care issues, including ACP.[27] Understanding the personal barriers that patients experience related to ACP is important, as some barriers may be general (eg, fear of dying) while others may be specific aspects of ACP, such as communication or identifying a surrogate decision maker.

Table 4 shows barriers identified by older adults[6] and suggestions on how to approach them. The diverse barriers reflect the need for clinicians to explore each individual's perspective on ACP, as willingness to engage in ACP may be influenced by personal experiences and family, cultural, religious, or spiritual values. As barriers are identified, the clinician and other team members should work with the patient to offer targeted support.

Identifying Surrogate Decision Makers

Even with limited time, clinicians can emphasize the importance of choosing a trusted person as a surrogate decision maker. **Table 2** provides language to assist clinicians with promoting the choice of a surrogate and discussing the concept of flexibility in decision making. The surrogate needs to be asked to assume the responsibility and to agree to his or her role, and there needs to be communication and documentation of the surrogate as a medical power of attorney in the medical record.[26,28] In some cases, it may be appropriate for clinicians to facilitate a family meeting or conference call to assist patients in identifying and communicating their wishes with a surrogate and others they wish to be involved.

There are challenges with involving surrogate decision makers. For example, surrogates may incorrectly understand patients' values and preferences.[29] Clinicians can encourage patients and surrogates to have ongoing discussions over time as patients'

Table 3 Characteristics of advance care planning stages of change	
Stage of Change	**Description**
Precontemplation	Individual lacks awareness of or has no desire to engage in ACP
Contemplation of future care wishes and values	Individual understands the relevance of ACP their own lives and begins to form intentions to engage in ACP
Preparation	Values clarification and planning stage for actions related to ACP
Action	Engaging in the ACP process through doing an action, such as: • Discussions with family or friends • Discussion with clinicians • Advance directive documentation (ie, medical power of attorney, living will)
Maintenance	Reflecting on choices and evolving values, revising advance directive documents accordingly

Adapted from Refs.[6,25,28,31]

Table 4	
Potential barriers to advance care planning and general suggestions for clinicians	
Barriers Identified by Patients[6,27]	Suggestions for Overcoming Barriers
Too difficult to think about dying	Empathic and reflective listening
Lack of knowledge	Ask permission to discuss ACP specifically,
Inability to plan for the future because of	including arranging specific clinic visit time
challenging current life/social issues	Refer to a social worker to assist with unmet
Planning not necessary because of the	social/financial needs
assumption that family/doctors know what	Refer to chaplain, behavioral health, or
to do, or there are no medical choices to be	bereavement or other community-based
made	support resources
Future in God's hands	Invite family to clinic visit
Suffering is necessary	Address depression, grief, or losses
Physician will make decisions	Recommend an ACP decision tool
Lack of available surrogate decision maker	Provide health education in easy-to-read
Putting things down in writing might result	format
in treatment being withdrawn too soon	Consider health navigators[51] or trained
Loved ones unable or unwilling to discuss	facilitators[3] (ie, Respecting Choices
ACP	program)
Educational materials are too difficult to	
understand	

values may change. Despite these problems, the authors believe that surrogates are generally beneficial, particularly when they are able to provide illustrations of patients' life stories to inform medical decision making.[30]

Asking About Values Related to Quality of Life

Clinicians should initiate conversations that help patients articulate their values related to medical options and quality of life, especially in the setting of serious illness. **Table 2** provides questions to help individuals describe what quality of life means to them, consider their attitudes or preferences toward life-sustaining treatments, and reflect on trade-offs between quality of life and quantity of life.[31] Individuals can articulate values over time to guide decisions, including discussing whether certain health states would make life not worth living. Even when older adults have advance directive documents, many individuals have not had substantive conversations about their values and often have not considered how their values may be influenced by likely future medical circumstances, given their illnesses. Clinicians can teach older adults to ask questions to help make informed medical decisions based on identified values (eg, "What are the risks? What are the benefits? What are the burdens?").

Documenting Advance Care Planning Preferences

Clinicians have 2 major roles in supporting the documentation of ACP preferences. First, clinicians need access to advance directive forms to enable patients to formally identify a surrogate decision maker (ie, medical power of attorney) or preferences for future medical care (ie, living will). The American Bar Association has developed a Consumer's Toolkit for Health Care Advance Planning that includes a free, nearly universal Power of Attorney for Health Care form and links to state-specific forms.[32] Baseline knowledge of each form is important, including content and state-specific requirements for witnesses or notarization. Clinicians should emphasize the importance of discussing the contents and sharing copies, especially with surrogates. Second, in the medical record, clinicians should document the content of ACP discussions and communicate with other health care team members. Advance directive copies should be officially added to the medical record. Ideally the medical record, whether electronic or paper, has specific mechanisms to highlight ACP discussions and documents promote easy retrieval and updating both across and outside of the patient's health care system.[33]

Translating Preferences into Medical Care Plans

Translation of individual preferences into medical orders that direct medical treatments is especially important in the care of older adults with serious illness or frequent care transitions. Out-of-hospital medical orders, variously called POLST, Medical Orders for Scope of Treatment (MOST), or other names, serve as legally approved forms to document and communicate specific life-sustaining treatment wishes of seriously ill patients.[34] Clinicians will frequently need to translate preferences or advance directives into a medical care plan if appropriate in the context of the patient's current medical condition. Examples of common treatment planning that involves translation of the patient's values and existing advance directives include:

- General scope of care options: life-prolonging (ie, CPR and life-sustaining treatments), limited interventions (ie, hospitalization with limitations in the extent of medical intervention), or comfort care (ie, symptom relief)[34,35]
- Role of artificial nutrition and hydration
- Role of hospitalization and/or outpatient services such as hospice[11]
- Role of CPR, including recommending for or against this procedure[36]

Table 2 provides examples for talking with older adults and translating preferences into current medical care plans, such as CPR directives, do-not-resuscitate orders, and out-of-hospital medical orders. Specifically, clinicians can use POLST forms to translate ACP preferences into medical orders, including CPR, scope of treatment, artificial nutrition by tube, and, in some states, antibiotic use, based on conversations with patients or surrogates.[37] As they generally limit medical interventions, these orders are primarily used in patients with advanced illnesses and limited life expectancies. These medical orders are legal documents that should be followed in any setting (ie, home, hospital, and nursing home).

SPECIAL CONSIDERATIONS FOR ADVANCE CARE PLANNING IN THE ELDERLY

As clinicians and the outpatient care team undertake ACP, there are special considerations to account for in the older adult, such as:

- Presence of cognitive impairment, suggesting the need to assess decision-making capacity[38] related to ACP and to involve surrogates if available
- Living apart from a potential surrogates (ie, long-distance family member)
- Lack of available surrogates owing to absent or fractured relationships or the death of loved ones
- Prior ACP, especially advance directives that are no longer accurate or accessible
- Multiple health care providers related to multiple medical conditions and/or care transitions resulting in a fragmented ACP process
- Need for hearing aids, pocket talkers, and/or glasses because of sensory impairments

TEAM-BASED APPROACHES TO ADVANCE CARE PLANNING

As patients engage in ACP, clinicians and the outpatient care team can work together to support ongoing values: clarification discussions; education and counseling about risks, benefits, and burdens of medical treatment options; and communication with patients, surrogates, and the health care system as patients' health status, needs, and preferences change over time. The multidisciplinary team can use the key concepts as guides to identify how patients may have engaged in ACP or brief counseling opportunities that they can help with (**Box 2**).

Clinicians and the outpatient care team can seek to address clinical and health care system barriers to ACP by systematically identifying barriers and incorporating ACP over multiple visits. A structured, systems-based approach can be used to identify opportunities for improvement.[39,40] Existing clinic programs can be modified to support ACP. For example, ACP interventions (ie, counseling, education, support, and patient-centered ACP tools [see next section]) could be added to existing programs that address other behavioral health needs, such as tobacco cessation or chronic disease management; or routine preventive care, such as the Medicare Annual Wellness visits and programs related to maintaining healthy lives as older adults (ie, driving, exercise, nutrition). Alternatively, the team could systematically incorporate the use of patient-centered ACP tools to help prepare patients before they come into the office to partake in these conversations.

NEW PATIENT-CENTERED ADVANCE CARE PLANNING TOOLS

Recent advances in ACP include the development of accessible tools to assist patients with knowledge and decision making related to ACP. Because ACP can be a personnel-intensive and time-intensive process, helping patients and families begin this process on their own is useful. In a randomized controlled trial, a patient-completed preference form increased ACP communication from 11% to 30%.[41] Although not all tools have been formally tested in research settings, various tools offer practical benefit for patients and their families.[42]

- PREPARE (https://www.prepareforyourcare.org/)[43] is an ACP Web site with videos that focuses on preparing patients for communication and decision making.
- ACP Decisions (http://www.acpdecisions.org/) presents ACP videos describing how overall goals of care, CPR, and mechanical ventilation can influence patients' and surrogates' preferences for end-of-life care.[35,44]
- The Conversation Project (http://theconversationproject.org/)[45] provides a written toolkit with values-based questions to help individuals start ACP conversations.
- The GO WISH Card Game,[46] a set of cards that describe potential quality-of-life values, may facilitate conversations among older adults with cognitive impairment.

Box 2
Examples of multidisciplinary team-based approaches to ACP

- Front-desk staff can ask patients to bring advance directives to clinic, inform the clinician, document their presence, and copy for medical record
- Medical assistant can prescreen the medical record for evidence of prior ACP and highlight the opportunity for the clinician to initiate/update during visit
- Staff member with ACP counseling training can ask about prior ACP, especially potential surrogate decision makers, and document and communicate for the clinician to follow up

- Making your Wishes Known (https://www.makingyourwishesknown.com/)[47,48] and MyDirectives (https://mydirectives.com/)[49] are tailored Web sites that provide video instructions and explanations to complete advance directives.

SUMMARY

Clinicians who care for older adults can engage older adults in ACP through multiple brief discussions over time. ACP emphasizes choosing a surrogate decision maker, identifying personal values, communicating values and preferences with surrogates and clinicians, documenting preferences for future medical care, and appointing a surrogate decision maker in advance directives in addition to, when appropriate, translating preferences into specific medical treatment plans or medical orders. While older adults, clinicians, and health care systems face specific needs and barriers related to ACP, multidisciplinary teams can incorporate key ACP concepts into brief clinic visits. In addition, several patient-centered ACP tools are available to support ACP in the outpatient setting.

REFERENCES

1. Schneiderman LJ, Kronick R, Kaplan RM, et al. Effects of offering advance directives on medical treatments and costs. Ann Intern Med 1992;117(7):599–606.
2. Silveira MJ, Kim SY, Langa KM. Advance directives and outcomes of surrogate decision making before death. N Engl J Med 2010;362(13):1211–8.
3. Hammes BJ, Rooney BL. Death and end-of-life planning in one Midwestern community. Arch Intern Med 1998;158(4):383–90.
4. Detering KM, Hancock AD, Reade MC, et al. The impact of advance care planning on end of life care in elderly patients: randomised controlled trial. BMJ 2010; 340:c1345.
5. Bischoff KE, Sudore R, Miao Y, et al. Advance care planning and the quality of end-of-life care in older adults. J Am Geriatr Soc 2013;61(2):209–14.
6. Fried TR, Bullock K, Iannone L, et al. Understanding advance care planning as a process of health behavior change. J Am Geriatr Soc 2009;57(9):1547–55.
7. Tierney WM, Dexter PR, Gramelspacher GP, et al. The effect of discussions about advance directives on patients' satisfaction with primary care. J Gen Intern Med 2001;16(1):32–40.
8. Wright AA, Zhang B, Ray A, et al. Associations between end-of-life discussions, patient mental health, medical care near death, and caregiver bereavement adjustment. JAMA 2008;300(14):1665–73.
9. Fromme EK, Zive D, Schmidt TA, et al. Association between physician orders for life-sustaining treatment for scope of treatment and in-hospital death in Oregon. J Am Geriatr Soc 2014;62(7):1246–51.
10. Nicholas LH, Langa KM, Iwashyna TJ, et al. Regional variation in the association between advance directives and end-of-life Medicare expenditures. JAMA 2011; 306(13):1447–53.
11. Ache K, Harrold J, Harris P, et al. Are advance directives associated with better hospice care? J Am Geriatr Soc 2014;62(6):1091–6.
12. Kirchhoff KT, Hammes BJ, Kehl KA, et al. Effect of a disease-specific advance care planning intervention on end-of-life care. J Am Geriatr Soc 2012;60(5):946–50.
13. Hammes BJ, Rooney BL, Gundrum JD. A comparative, retrospective, observational study of the prevalence, availability, and specificity of advance care plans in a county that implemented an advance care planning microsystem. J Am Geriatr Soc 2010;58(7):1249–55.

14. Hickman SE, Nelson CA, Perrin NA, et al. A comparison of methods to communicate treatment preferences in nursing facilities: traditional practices versus the physician orders for life-sustaining treatment program. J Am Geriatr Soc 2010;58(7):1241–8.
15. Tolle SW, Tilden VP, Nelson CA, et al. A prospective study of the efficacy of the physician order form for life-sustaining treatment. J Am Geriatr Soc 1998;46(9):1097–102.
16. Teno J, Lynn J, Wenger N, et al. Advance directives for seriously ill hospitalized patients: effectiveness with the patient self-determination act and the SUPPORT intervention. SUPPORT investigators. Study to understand prognoses and preferences for outcomes and risks of treatment. J Am Geriatr Soc 1997;45(4):500–7.
17. Covinsky KE, Fuller JD, Yaffe K, et al. Communication and decision-making in seriously ill patients: findings of the SUPPORT project. The study to understand prognoses and preferences for outcomes and risks of treatments. J Am Geriatr Soc 2000;48(5 Suppl):S187–93.
18. Teno JM, Gruneir A, Schwartz Z, et al. Association between advance directives and quality of end-of-life care: a national study. J Am Geriatr Soc 2007;55(2):189–94.
19. Silveira MJ, Wiitala W, Piette J. Advance directive completion by elderly Americans: a decade of change. J Am Geriatr Soc 2014;62(4):706–10.
20. Heyland DK, Barwich D, Pichora D, et al. Failure to engage hospitalized elderly patients and their families in advance care planning. JAMA Intern Med 2013;173(9):778–87.
21. Ahluwalia SC, Bekelman DB, Huynh AK, et al. Barriers and strategies to an iterative model of advance care planning communication. Am J Hosp Palliat Care 2014. [Epub ahead of print].
22. Ahluwalia SC, Levin JR, Lorenz KA, et al. Missed opportunities for advance care planning communication during outpatient clinic visits. J Gen Intern Med 2012;27(4):445–51.
23. McMahan RD, Knight SJ, Fried TR, et al. Advance care planning beyond advance directives: perspectives from patients and surrogates. J Pain Symptom Manage 2013;46(3):355–65.
24. Spoelhof GD, Elliott B. Implementing advance directives in office practice. Am Fam Physician 2012;85(5):461–6.
25. Sudore RL, Schickedanz AD, Landefeld CS, et al. Engagement in multiple steps of the advance care planning process: a descriptive study of diverse older adults. J Am Geriatr Soc 2008;56(6):1006–13.
26. Sudore RL, Fried TR. Redefining the "planning" in advance care planning: preparing for end-of-life decision making. Ann Intern Med 2010;153(4):256–61.
27. Schickedanz AD, Schillinger D, Landefeld CS, et al. A clinical framework for improving the advance care planning process: start with patients' self-identified barriers. J Am Geriatr Soc 2009;57(1):31–9.
28. Sudore RL, Stewart AL, Knight SJ, et al. Development and validation of a questionnaire to detect behavior change in multiple advance care planning behaviors. PLoS One 2013;8(9):e72465.
29. Shalowitz DI, Garrett-Mayer E, Wendler D. The accuracy of surrogate decision makers: a systematic review. Arch Intern Med 2006;166(5):493–7.
30. Sulmasy DP, Snyder L. Substituted interests and best judgments: an integrated model of surrogate decision making. JAMA 2010;304(17):1946–7.
31. Fried TR, Redding CA, Robbins ML, et al. Stages of change for the component behaviors of advance care planning. J Am Geriatr Soc 2010;58(12):2329–36.

32. American Bar Association, Commission on Law and Aging. Consumer's toolkit for health care planning. 2014. Available at: http://www.americanbar.org/groups/law_aging/resources/health_care_decision_making/consumer_s_toolkit_for_health_care_advance_planning.html. Accessed August 9, 2014.

33. Wilson CJ, Newman J, Tapper S, et al. Multiple locations of advance care planning documentation in an electronic health record: are they easy to find? J Palliat Med 2013;16(9):1089–94.

34. Physicians Orders for Life-Sustaining Treatment (POLST) paradigm. Available at: http://www.polst.org/. Accessed July 26, 2014.

35. Volandes AE, Brandeis GH, Davis AD, et al. A randomized controlled trial of a goals-of-care video for elderly patients admitted to skilled nursing facilities. J Palliat Med 2012;15(7):805–11.

36. Blinderman CD, Krakauer EL, Solomon MZ. Time to revise the approach to determining cardiopulmonary resuscitation status. JAMA 2012;307(9):917–8.

37. Fromme EK, Zive D, Schmidt TA, et al. Registry do-not-resuscitate orders and other patient treatment preferences. JAMA 2012;307(1):34–5.

38. Sessums LL, Zembrzuska H, Jackson JL. Does this patient have medical decision-making capacity? JAMA 2011;306(4):420–7.

39. Grol R. Improving patient care: the implementation of change in health care. 2nd edition. Chichester (United Kingdom): Wiley Blackwell; 2013.

40. Chaudoir SR, Dugan AG, Barr CH. Measuring factors affecting implementation of health innovations: a systematic review of structural, organizational, provider, patient, and innovation level measures. Implement Sci 2013;8:22.

41. Au DH, Udris EM, Engelberg RA, et al. A randomized trial to improve communication about end-of-life care among patients with COPD. Chest 2012;141(3):726–35.

42. Butler M, Ratner E, McCreedy E, et al. Decision aids for advance care planning: an overview of the state of the science. Ann Intern Med 2014;161(6):408–18.

43. Sudore RL, Knight SJ, McMahan RD, et al. A novel website to prepare diverse older adults for decision making and advance care planning: a pilot study. J Pain Symptom Manage 2013;47(4):674–86.

44. Volandes AE, Mitchell SL, Gillick MR, et al. Using video images to improve the accuracy of surrogate decision-making: a randomized controlled trial. J Am Med Dir Assoc 2009;10(8):575–80.

45. The Conversation Project. Available at: http://theconversationproject.org/starter-kit/intro/. Accessed October 13, 2012.

46. Lankarani-Fard A, Knapp H, Lorenz KA, et al. Feasibility of discussing end-of-life care goals with inpatients using a structured, conversational approach: the go wish card game. J Pain Symptom Manage 2010;39(4):637–43.

47. Green MJ, Levi BH. Development of an interactive computer program for advance care planning. Health Expect 2009;12(1):60–9.

48. Making Your Wishes Known. Available at: https://www.makingyourwishesknown.com/. Accessed July 26, 2014.

49. MyDirectives. Online advance medical directives, better than a living will. Available at: https://mydirectives.com/. Accessed July 26, 2014.

50. Goldhirsch S, Chai E, Meier D, et al. Geriatric palliative care. New York: Oxford University Press; 2014.

51. Fischer SM, Sauaia A, Kutner JS. Patient navigation: a culturally competent strategy to address disparities in palliative care. J Palliat Med 2007;10(5):1023–8.

Urinary Incontinence and Pelvic Organ Prolapse

Kirk M. Anderson, MD[a], Karlotta Davis, MD, MPH[b], Brian J. Flynn, MD[a],*

KEYWORDS

- Urinary incontinence • Stress urinary incontinence • Urinary urge incontinence
- Pelvic organ prolapse • Geriatric assessment • Urinary tract disorders

KEY POINTS

- Urinary continence and pelvic organ prolapse in the elderly is widely prevalent and significantly affects quality of life. The primary care physician should ask about urinary incontinence in all geriatric patients.
- Accurate characterization of type of incontinence and prolapse is essential in forming an appropriate treatment plan.
- Behavioral and lifestyle modification is the cornerstone in treatment for stress, urgency, and functional incontinence.
- Frail elderly require special attention to avoid complications of urinary incontinence and prolapse. Care should be delivered with a multidisciplinary team-based approach.

INTRODUCTION

Urinary incontinence (UI) as defined by the International Continence Society is the complaint of any involuntary leakage of urine.[1] Urinary incontinence affects approximately 36% of women older than 60 years and 11% to 16% of men older than 65 in the United States.[2,3] An increase in UI prevalence with age is caused by multiple factors including increased incidence of comorbidities such as obesity and diabetes, polypharmacy, and age-related cognitive and functional decline. Urinary incontinence in the community and care facility setting is a significant economic burden with as estimated $19.5 billion spent in 2000 on the care of incontinence.[4] Pelvic organ prolapse (POP) can occur concomitantly with urinary incontinence. It can significantly affect quality of life in women of all ages. It is estimated that 3% and 4.1% of women age 60 to 79 and greater than 80, respectively, are affected by POP.[5]

~ 20 billion
y2k

Disclosures: None.
[a] Division of Urology, Department of Surgery, University of Colorado Denver, Academic Office One Building, 12631 East 17th Avenue, Box C319, Room L15-5602, Aurora, CO 80045, USA;
[b] Department of Obstetrics and Gynecology, Division of Female Pelvic Medicine and Reconstructive Surgery, University of Colorado Denver, 12631 East 17th Avenue, Room 4208, B198-2, Aurora, CO 80045, USA
* Corresponding author.
E-mail address: Brian.Flynn@UCdenver.edu

http://dx.doi.org/10.1016/j.mcna.2014.11.011
0025-7125/15/$ – see front matter © 2015 Elsevier Inc. All rights reserved.
medical.theclinics.com

Lower urinary tract function is dependent on 2 basic processes: the ability to fill or store urine and the ability to empty urine. In the absence of filling-phase dysfunction, the bladder is able to accommodate an increasing volume of urine at low pressures. This must occur in the absence of involuntary bladder contraction with adequate bladder outlet resistance to avoid unwanted leakage of urine. Normal emptying requires a coordinated contraction of detrusor muscle with a simultaneous decrease in outlet resistance provided by the voluntary and involuntary sphincter mechanisms. Lower urinary tract dysfunction can be broadly categorized as failure to fill or store or empty owing to failure of the bladder, bladder outlet, or a combination (**Fig. 1**). Urinary incontinence can result from a failure of either of these mechanisms or a combination. Urinary incontinence is categorized as outlined in **Table 1**.

This article reviews the diagnosis and medical management of urinary incontinence and prolapse in the outpatient primary care setting. Conditions that should prompt referral to a surgical specialist are also briefly discussed.

INITIAL EVALUATION OF URINARY INCONTINENCE AND PELVIC ORGAN PROLAPSE

The initial evaluation in primary care should include a careful history, physical examination, and urinalysis. A thorough history can aid in distinguishing between the different types of incontinence, although this can be difficult in elderly patients with cognitive decline. Correctly identifying the type of urinary dysfunction is important when considering management options, although many patients will have a combination of symptoms (**Table 2**). Additionally, it is important to determine if the UI is acute or an established condition. Acute incontinence is typically a result of an acute change that, once corrected, may resolve the incontinence. Consideration should be given to various conditions that cause incontinence that may prompt referral to a surgical specialist after the initial visit (**Table 3**). Microscopic ($\geq$3 red blood cells per high-power field on microscopy) or gross hematuria, rectal or prostatic mass, palpable bladder, and failure of initial therapies should also prompt referral to a specialist (**Fig. 2**).

Similar to UI, POP should be initially evaluated with a careful history and physical examination. A thorough history can aid in distinguishing between the different types of prolapse. The most common prolapse complaint is the awareness of a vaginal

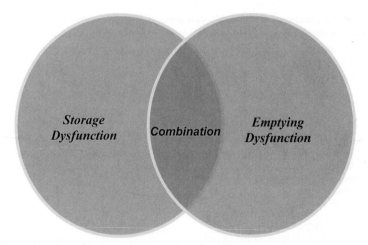

Fig. 1. Categorization of lower urinary tract dysfunction.

Table 1	
Types of urinary incontinence	
Stress incontinence	The complaint of involuntary leakage on effort or exertion or on sneezing or coughing
Urge incontinence	The complaint of involuntary leakage accompanied by or immediately preceded by urgency
Mixed incontinence	Combination of stress and urge incontinence
Overflow incontinence	Involuntary leakage of urine from a bladder at or near volume capacity in the absence of detrusor contraction
Functional incontinence	Leakage of urine in the presence of physical or cognitive deficits and in the absence of urinary system pathologic abnormality

bulge, fullness, or pressure. These indicators are owing to prolapse of the bladder (cystocele), rectum (rectocele), or uterus (uterine prolapse). Patients with a cystocele will frequently complain of difficulty emptying the bladder, urinary urgency, incomplete emptying, and, rarely, urinary retention. Patients with a rectocele will complain of difficulty with fecal evacuation and the need to splint to have a bowel movement. Constipation may cause or be the result of a rectocele. Correctly identifying the type of prolapse is important when considering management options. Failure of initial therapies should also prompt referral to a specialist.

The evaluation in a specialist's office will include components of the initial evaluation and use of validated questionnaires, pad test to determine degree of incontinence, bladder log (voiding diary), and assessment of postvoid residual. Cystoscopy and urodynamic testing may be indicated in more complex cases to characterize the type of incontinence and direct overall treatment goals of both the patient and caregiver if applicable.

CLASSIFICATION AND TREATMENT OF URINARY INCONTINENCE

Urinary incontinence is typically classified as stress, urge, overflow, or functional incontinence. As previously stated, successful treatment is dependent on correctly identifying the type of incontinence. Regardless of the type of incontinence, most patients will initially use diapers or urinary pads. Although effective at allowing patients to maintain dryness, pad usage is costly and can affect quality of life because of the need for frequent changes and odor. For the frail elderly with limited mobility, infrequent pad or diaper changes can lead to skin breakdown and complex wounds. Caregivers should be educated on the importance of frequent diaper/pad changes to limit the risk of skin complications.

Table 2	
Common symptoms of lower urinary tract dysfunction	
Storage Dysfunction	**Emptying Dysfunction**
Urinary frequency	Hesitancy
Urinary urgency	Straining
Nocturia	Urinary retention
UUI	Urinary frequency
SUI	

Table 3 Differential diagnosis to consider referral to specialist	
Local Pathology	**Female Factors**
Bladder calculi	Vaginal atrophy
Bladder tumor	Vesicovaginal fistula
Metabolic Factors	**Male Factors**
Diabetes	Benign prostatic hypertrophy
Polydipsia	Prostate cancer

ACUTE INCONTINENCE

Acute onset of incontinence is typically caused by conditions separate from pathologic or anatomic changes in the genitourinary system. The most common causes can be remembered with the pneumonic "DIAPERS" (**Box 1**). Once the underlying cause of delirium is treated, UI typically resolves. Infection is a cause of acute incontinence and can be diagnosed based on symptoms, urinalysis, and urine culture. Prescribing antibiotics in the setting of asymptomatic bacteriuria should be avoided, as this can result in adverse effects of antimicrobial medications and increase the probability of developing drug-resistant microbial isolates in the future.[6] The optimal duration of antibiotics for an uncomplicated urinary tract infection is unknown. A

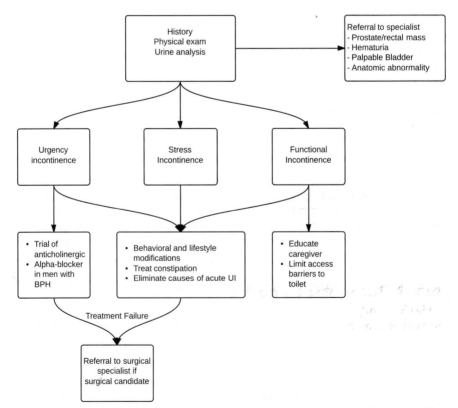

Fig. 2. Urinary incontinence management algorithm. BPH, benign prostatic hypertrophy.

Box 1
Causes of acute urinary incontinence
Delirium
Infection
Alcohol
Pharmaceuticals
Excess urine production
Reduced mobility
Stool impaction

Cochrane review found no difference in clinical failure rates when comparing a 3- to 6-day course of antibiotics with a 7- to 14-day course in older women with uncomplicated urinary tract infection. Thus, a shorter course in such patients is recommended to limit adverse effects of a prolonged course of antimicrobials.[7]

Alcohol and pharmaceuticals can also contribute to urinary incontinence by various mechanisms of action (**Table 4**). Excess urine production can also precipitate UI. Increasing volume of urine can be a result of increased urine production caused by diuretic medications, excessive fluid consumption, and glucosuria. Additionally, conditions such as congenital heart failure, peripheral venous insufficiency, and hypoalbuminia/malnourishment can cause fluid retention that can result in excess urine production. These conditions often occur in combination, and medical optimization of each can reduce high volumes of urine production that may be precipitating UI. Restricted mobility will be discussed further in the section covering functional incontinence. Finally, constipation is a risk factor for both transient and chronic urinary incontinence.[8] It is present in approximately one-third of people 60 years and older.[9] In a cohort of women age 65 to 89 years with lower urinary tract symptoms and constipation, treatment of constipation resulted in decreased rates of urinary frequency and urgency and reduced postvoid residual urine volume.[10]

STRESS URINARY INCONTINENCE

Stress urinary incontinence (SUI) is the involuntary leakage of urine during activities that increase intra-abdominal pressure such as straining, lifting, or coughing. Stress incontinence is uncommon in men with the exception of men who have had surgical therapy of the prostate for benign or malignant disease. In women, stress incontinence occurs primarily because of urethral hypermobility and intrinsic sphincter deficiency.

Table 4	
Medications and mechanisms of action affecting continence	
Mechanism of Action	**Class of Medication**
Increased urine production	Diuretics, thiazolidinediones, calcium channel blockers, some anticonvulsants (latter 3 medications for fluid retention)
Sedation/immobility	Sedative hypnotics, antipsychotics, some antidepressants, opiates
Increased bladder outlet resistance and/or inhibited bladder contractility	α-adrenergic agonists, anticholinergics, opioids, muscle relaxants

Treatment of Stress Urinary Incontinence

Self-care, also known as lifestyle modification, should be the cornerstone of nonoperative management of UI. For example weight loss, smoking cessation, and avoidance of triggers are simple nonoperative measures that can be effective in the motivated patient. Obesity increases the risk of developing stress incontinence.[11] In a randomized controlled trial of women with a mean body mass index of 36 and urinary incontinence, a 6-month diet and exercise program resulting in weight loss significantly decreased the frequency of self-reported UI episodes.[12]

If self-care is ineffective, pelvic floor muscle training (PFMT), commonly referred to as Kegel exercises, has been shown to improve the volume of leakage and number of incontinent episodes in older men and women.[13,14] Although the exact mechanism by which improving strength of pelvic floor musculature improves continence is not clear, there is sufficient evidence that PMFT is an important component of nonoperative management of SUI. The optimal regimen of PFMT has not been determined; however, the slight variation in techniques is less important in improving results than maintaining a regular schedule of pelvic floor exercise. A suggested exercise regimen is shown in **Box 2**. As with many lifestyle modifications programs, ensuring continued adherence to the PMFT program is challenging. In a review of women 15 years after the end of a formal PMFT program, only 28% maintained exercise at least on a weekly basis.[15] The clinician should encourage the patient to incorporate PMFT into a daily routine and ask at scheduled visits about adherence to their exercise program.

Another form of nonsurgical treatment of SUI in women is the vaginal pessary. Although primarily used for pelvic organ prolapse, pessaries are found to improve stress incontinence in women.[16] Appropriate device and size selection is important to optimize outcome. Care should be taken in the elderly population, as adequate dexterity and cognitive function are essential to care for the device to avoid devastating complications from the neglected pessary.

In patients do not respond to nonsurgical therapy or those who are not motivated to adhere to PMFT, there are several surgical options. Surgical therapy in women typically includes bulking agents, colposuspension, and slings. In women fit for surgery who are older than 70, slings are found to significantly improve continence and patient-reported quality of life.[17,18] Surgical therapy in men for SUI also includes bulking agents and slings and artificial urinary sphincter placement for more severe cases.

Box 2
Suggested pelvic floor muscle training and bladder training techniques

Pelvic floor muscle training

- Contraction of pelvic floor muscle group for 2–10 seconds (maximum duration possible, with progressive goal of 10–15 second contraction)
- Sets of 10 pelvic floor muscle contractions — ?. set = 3 sets or just 1 T10 (vs 3 T10) I think latter
- Repeat 3 times/d

Bladder training

- Scheduled voiding with increasing intervals between voids to goal
- Fixed interval voiding (in setting of pure stress incontinence to reduce bladder volume)
- Urge inhibition techniques (meditation, distraction techniques, prompted pelvic floor contraction)

URGENCY INCONTINENCE

Urinary urgency is the sudden compelling desire to void that is difficult to defer. When this symptom coexists with incontinence, it is referred to as urge urinary incontinence (UUI). Differences between SUI and UUI are outlined in **Table 5**. Overactive bladder is the symptom complex of urinary urgency with frequency or nocturia with or without incontinence. Normal bladder filling and storage is a result of complex interaction between the cellular components of the bladder and the central and peripheral nervous system that innervate and control voiding. Disruption of these components can affect normal filling and result in unwanted bladder contraction and resultant UI. Management options of UUI consists of behavioral and lifestyle modification, pharmacologic treatment, and surgery.

Treatment of Urgency Incontinence

Behavioral and lifestyle modification is the cornerstone in the initial management of UUI (**Fig. 3**). The relationship between diet and urinary incontinence is not well established. Limiting alcohol intake and reducing caffeine intake to less than 200 mg/d (<2 cups of regular coffee) is suggested to reduce symptoms of urgency, although the effects on incontinence are unknown.[19] Pelvic floor muscle training may reduce episodes of urgency incontinence; however, the benefits are less clear when compared with improving SUI. Bladder training (see **Box 2**) should also be a component of lifestyle modification, although there are limited data showing significant improvement.[20] Bladder training and pelvic floor muscle training should be done in combination when possible to reduce episodes of UUI.[21]

Pharmacologic management of UUI consists primarily of anticholinergic medications that block the effects of acetylcholine on the muscarinic receptors in the bladder. Several antimuscarinic medications are available (**Table 6**) and data are insufficient to suggest greater clinical efficacy for any one anticholinergic. These agents are generally well tolerated but can cause significant dry mouth and constipation and are contraindicated in patients with closed-angle glaucoma. There have been reports of impaired cognition with anticholinergic medications; however, this is uncommon. Immediate-release oral oxybutynin in doses greater than 10 mg/d has been associated with significant cognitive decline; however, in doses less than 10 mg/d the cognitive side-effect profile is similar to that of other antimuscarinics. Anticholinergics should be used with caution in patients with Alzheimer's disease or in those taking an acetylcholinesterase inhibitors because of risk of acute worsening of dementia and delusions.[22] Additionally, caution should be exercised in elderly patients with elevated postvoid residual (PVR) urine volume. There is no well-established PVR above which initiating an anticholinergic medication is absolutely contraindicated, although caution

| Table 5 | | |
| Differences between stress and urgency incontinence | | |
Symptoms	**Urgency Incontinence**	**Stress Incontinence**
Urgency	Yes	No
Frequency	Yes	No
Leakage with activity	No	Yes
Amount leaked with incontinence episode	Large	Small/moderate
Ability to reach toilet in time with urge to void	No	Yes
Waking to void at night	Usually	Seldom

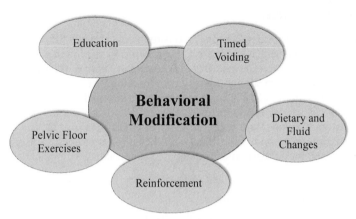

Fig. 3. Behavioral and lifestyle modification principles.

should be exercised when PVR is greater than 150 mL. After initiating treatment with an antimuscarinic in patients with an elevated PVR, it should be periodically monitored to ensure adequate bladder emptying.

Mirabegron was recently introduced as an alternative to anticholinergics. It is a β-3 adrenergic receptor agonist and avoids the classic anticholinergic side effects such as dry mouth, dry eyes, and constipation. The β-3 adrenergic receptor in the bladder wall is normally stimulated by norepinephrine in the sympathetic pathway promoting bladder relaxation during filling. This is a new class of medication that is promising in the treatment of urinary urgency and UUI. It is found to be effective and well tolerated in patients older than 65 years with 1 year of follow-up.[23]

In patients with UUI refractory to lifestyle modification and pharmacologic therapy, referral to a specialist is recommended. Surgical options for UUI include intravesical injection of botulinium A toxin, percutaneous tibial nerve stimulation, and sacral nerve stimulation and, in the most severe cases, bladder augmentation and urinary diversion.

Table 6
Medications for treatment of urinary urgency and urgency incontinence

	Common Dosing
Anticholinergic Medications	
Oxybutynin (immediate release, extended release oral, patch, gel)	2.5–5 mg PO BID-TID 5–15 mg PO qd 1 patch (3.9 mg/d) q 3 d 10% gel topically once daily
Tolterodine (immediate release, extended release)	1–2 mg PO BID 2–4 mg PO qd
Darifenacin	7.5 mg-15 mg PO qd
Solifenacin	5–10 mg PO qd
Trospium (immediate release, extended release)	20 mg PO BID 60 mg PO qd
Fesoterodine	4–8 mg PO qd
β-3 adrenergic agonist	
Mirabegron	25–50 mg PO qd

OVERFLOW INCONTINENCE

Overflow incontinence is a result of failure to empty the bladder from bladder outlet obstruction or inadequate bladder contractility. In men, the most common etiology is bladder outlet obstruction from prostatic enlargement. In women, the most common etiology is an acontractile bladder. *- ? 2 ° —derys !*

Treatment of Overflow Incontinence

In the acute setting, this should be managed with placement of a urethral catheter as urine retention can cause acute kidney injury. Clean intermittent catheterization (CIC) is preferred over continuous catheterization to lower the risk of urinary tract infection.[24] However, in many elderly patients with retention, CIC is not practical because of impairments in cognitive and physical skills. In this setting, an indwelling urethral or suprapubic catheter may be more appropriate. In men and women with overflow incontinence, referral to a specialist is recommended.

FUNCTIONAL INCONTINENCE

Functional incontinence is the term to describe UI in the presence of physical or cognitive deficits and in the absence of urinary system pathologic abnormality. It is commonly diagnosed in the frail elderly. However, functional impairment should be considered a risk factor for other types of incontinence, as most elderly patients with a diagnosis of functional incontinence also have underlying stress, urge, or mixed incontinence.[25] Identifying functional barriers to normal voiding is an important part of minimizing UI. In the acute setting, such as after hip fracture, barriers to toilet use should be minimized. Use of bedside commode, condom catheters in men, and timing of fluid intake to coincide with availability of caregivers may improve the immobile patient's ability to remain dry. Additionally, having caregivers available for toilet assistance can prevent episodes of incontinence.[26]

INCONTINENCE IN THE FRAIL ELDERLY

Incontinence in elderly persons who require assistance for activities of daily living can adversely affect the patient's overall health and quality of life and that of the caregiver. An estimated 65% of nursing home residents have UI, and it is a leading cause for placement into a long-term care facility.[27] The International Consultation on Incontinence has issued guidelines for management of the frail elderly. Recommended lifestyle and behavioral modifications in this population are presented in **Table 7**. An important component is caregiver investment into the goals of improving continence.[28] The United States Center for Medicare and Medicaid services has issued guidelines on

Table 7	
Behavioral and lifestyle modifications in the frail elderly	
Prompted voiding	Prompting toilet use with contingent approval/praise Goal of increasing patient requested/self-initiated toilet use
Habit retraining	Use of bladder diary and identification of timing of voiding with goal of preempting incontinent episodes with planned toilet use
Timed voiding	Fixed interval toilet use in patients in absence of reinforcement or patient education
Combined toileting and exercise therapy	Physical exercise and pelvic floor training incorporating toilet mobility techniques

Table 8	
Stages of pelvic organ prolapse	
Stage 1	The most distal prolapse is more than 1 cm above the level of the hymen
Stage 2	The most distal prolapse is between 1 cm above and 1 cm below the hymen
Stage 3	The most distal prolapse is more than 1 cm below the hymen but no further than 2 cm less than TVL
Stage 4	Represents complete vault eversion; the most distal prolapse protrudes to at least TVL 2 cm

Abbreviation: TVL, total vaginal length.

urinary incontinence in the surveyor community; however, it has been questioned whether these guidelines have improved the quality of UI care in nursing home residents.[29,30]

CLASSIFICATION AND TREATMENT OF PELVIC ORGAN PROLAPSE

Pelvic organ prolapse is typically classified by prolapsing organ and stage (1–4) (**Table 8**).[31] Stages 3 and 4 prolapse usually cause symptoms, such as incomplete bladder empting, severe enough to warrant intervention. Regardless of the type of POP, most women will be candidates for nonoperative management. Lifestyle modifications to avoid triggers that increase intra-abdominal pressure, such as constipation, obesity, chronic cough, and lifting, should be eliminated. Similar to treatment for UI, PFMT is also effective in strengthening the pelvic floor and improving POP.[32] A pessary is a silicone device that is inserted into the vagina to provide support and improve symptoms of vaginal pressure and improve bladder emptying. Pessaries come in various shapes and sizes and need to be fitted properly to fit the patient's anatomy (**Fig. 4**). Proper fitting, education, and careful follow-up by a pelvic floor specialist are paramount in optimizing outcomes and avoiding a forgotten foreign body.

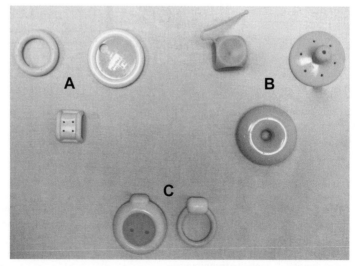

Fig. 4. Commonly used pessaries: Support (*A*), space filling (*B*), incontinence support (*C*).

SUMMARY

Urinary incontinence and pelvic organ prolapse are widely prevalent problems in the elderly population in both community and care facility settings. The primary care physician should be proactive in identifying UI and POP and engaging the patient and caregivers in a multimodal approach to management. Ancillary health care staff also serves as an important adjunct in sustaining improvements obtained through lifestyle and behavioral modifications. Referral to surgical specialists in the appropriate setting is an important component of the multidisciplinary approach that is necessary in achieving patient and caregiver goals.

REFERENCES

1. Abrams P, Cardozo L, Fall M, et al. The standardisation of terminology of lower urinary tract function: report from the standardisation sub-committee of the international continence society. Neurourol Urodyn 2002;21(2):167–78.
2. Dooley Y, Kenton K, Cao G, et al. Urinary incontinence prevalence: results from the National Health and Nutrition Examination Survey. J Urol 2008;179(2):656–61.
3. Markland AD, Goode PS, Redden DT, et al. Prevalence of urinary incontinence in men: results from the national health and nutrition examination survey. J Urol 2010;184(3):1022–7.
4. Hu TW, Wagner TH, Bentkover JD, et al. Costs of urinary incontinence and overactive bladder in the United States: a comparative study. Urology 2004;63(3): 461–5.
5. Nygaard I, Barber MD, Burgio KL, et al. Prevalence of symptomatic pelvic floor disorders in US women. JAMA 2008;300(11):1311–6.
6. Abrutyn E, Mossey J, Berlin JA, et al. Does asymptomatic bacteriuria predict mortality and does antimicrobial treatment reduce mortality in elderly ambulatory women? Ann Intern Med 1994;120(10):827–33.
7. Lutters M, Vogt-Ferrier NB. Antibiotic duration for treating uncomplicated, symptomatic lower urinary tract infections in elderly women. Cochrane Database Syst Rev 2008;(3):CD001535.
8. Carter D, Beer-Gabel M. Lower urinary tract symptoms in chronically constipated women. Int Urogynecol J 2012;23(12):1785–9.
9. American Gastroenterological Association, Bharucha AE, Dorn SD, et al. American Gastroenterological Association medical position statement on constipation. Gastroenterology 2013;144(1):211–7.
10. Charach G, Greenstein A, Rabinovich P, et al. Alleviating constipation in the elderly improves lower urinary tract symptoms. Gerontology 2001;47(2):72–6.
11. Osborn DJ, Strain M, Gomelsky A, et al. Obesity and female stress urinary incontinence. Urology 2013;82(4):759–63.
12. Subak LL, Wing R, West DS, et al. Weight loss to treat urinary incontinence in overweight and obese women. N Engl J Med 2009;360(5):481–90.
13. Sherburn M, Bird M, Carey M, et al. Incontinence improves in older women after intensive pelvic floor muscle training: an assessor-blinded randomized controlled trial. Neurourol Urodyn 2011;30(3):317–24.
14. Pereira VS, Escobar AC, Driusso P. Effects of physical therapy in older women with urinary incontinence: a systematic review. Rev Bras Fisioter 2012;16(6): 463–8.
15. Bo K, Kvarstein B, Nygaard I. Lower urinary tract symptoms and pelvic floor muscle exercise adherence after 15 years. Obstet Gynecol 2005;105(5 Pt 1): 999–1005.

16. Farrell SA, Singh B, Aldakhil L. Continence pessaries in the management of urinary incontinence in women. J Obstet Gynaecol Can 2004;26(2):113–7.

17. Carr LK, Walsh PJ, Abraham VE, et al. Favorable outcome of pubovaginal slings for geriatric women with stress incontinence. J Urol 1997;157(1):125–8.

18. Walsh K, Generao SE, White MJ, et al. The influence of age on quality of life outcome in women following a tension-free vaginal tape procedure. J Urol 2004;171(3):1185–8.

19. Wyman JF, Burgio KL, Newman DK. Practical aspects of lifestyle modifications and behavioural interventions in the treatment of overactive bladder and urgency urinary incontinence. Int J Clin Pract 2009;63(8):1177–91.

20. Wallace SA, Roe B, Williams K, et al. Bladder training for urinary incontinence in adults. Cochrane Database Syst Rev 2004;(1):CD001308.

21. Shamliyan TA, Kane RL, Wyman J, et al. Systematic review: randomized, controlled trials of nonsurgical treatments for urinary incontinence in women. Ann Intern Med 2008;148(6):459–73.

22. Pagoria D, O'Connor RC, Guralnick ML. Antimuscarinic drugs: review of the cognitive impact when used to treat overactive bladder in elderly patients. Curr Urol Rep 2011;12(5):351–7.

23. Wagg A, Cardozo L, Nitti VW, et al. The efficacy and tolerability of the beta3-adrenoceptor agonist mirabegron for the treatment of symptoms of overactive bladder in older patients. Age Ageing 2014;43(5):666–75.

24. Hooton TM, Bradley SF, Cardenas DD, et al. Diagnosis, prevention, and treatment of catheter-associated urinary tract infection in adults: 2009 International Clinical Practice Guidelines from the Infectious Diseases Society of America. Clin Infect Dis 2010;50(5):625–63.

25. Resnick NM, Yalla SV, Laurino E. The pathophysiology of urinary incontinence among institutionalized elderly persons. N Engl J Med 1989;320(1):1–7.

26. Gibbs CF, Johnson TM 2nd, Ouslander JG. Office management of geriatric urinary incontinence. Am J Med 2007;120(3):211–20.

27. Newman DK. Urinary incontinence, catheters, and urinary tract infections: an overview of CMS tag F 315. Ostomy Wound Manage 2006;52(12):34–6, 38, 40–4.

28. Booth J, Kumlien S, Zang Y. Promoting urinary continence with older people: key issues for nurses. Int J Older People Nurs 2009;4(1):63–9.

29. Surveyor Guidance for Incontinence and Catheters. State operations manual (SOM). Baltimore (MD): Department of Health & Human Services, Centers for Medicare & Medicaid Services. 2005.

30. DuBeau CE, Ouslander JG, Palmer MH. Knowledge and attitudes of nursing home staff and surveyors about the revised federal guidance for incontinence care. Gerontologist 2007;47(4):468–79.

31. Bump RC, Mattiasson A, Bo K, et al. The standardization of terminology of female pelvic organ prolapse and pelvic floor dysfunction. Am J Obstet Gynecol 1996; 175(1):10–7.

32. Braekken IH, Majida M, Engh ME, et al. Can pelvic floor muscle training reverse pelvic organ prolapse and reduce prolapse symptoms? An assessor-blinded, randomized, controlled trial. Am J Obstet Gynecol 2010;203(2):170.e1–7.

Antithrombotic Management of Atrial Fibrillation in the Elderly

Karli Edholm, MD[a], Nathan Ragle, MD[a],
Matthew T. Rondina, MD, MS[b,*]

KEYWORDS

- Anticoagulation • Atrial fibrillation • Elderly • Bleeding • Warfarin
- Antiplatelet agents • Risk stratification

KEY POINTS

- Older age remains one of the strongest risk factors for stroke in patients with atrial fibrillation (AF).
- Validated stroke risk stratification schemes, such as the $CHADS_2$ and CHA_2DS_2-VASc, should be used to estimate stroke risk and guide anticoagulation decisions in older adults with AF.
- Bleeding risk scores, such as HAS-BLED, should not be used to exclude patients from the use of oral anticoagulation (OAC) but rather to identify modifiable bleeding risk factors that can be managed to reduce a patient's risk of bleeding from anticoagulation.
- The significant decrease in intracranial bleeding risk with non–vitamin K oral anticoagulants (NOACs), combined with their fixed dosing schedules and fewer drug-drug interactions, provides potential advantages over vitamin K antagonists (VKAs) in older patients with AF.
- Antiplatelet agents should be reserved primarily for patients who are deemed unsuitable for, or refuse, OACs.

INTRODUCTION

OAC is the most effective way to prevent thromboembolic disease in patients with AF. For decades, aspirin and VKAs were the primary agents used to prevent thromboembolic disease in patients with AF. The approval of NOACs has now expanded the range

This work was supported by the National Institutes of Health and the National Institute on Aging (HL092161, AG040631, HL112311, and AG048022) and the University of Utah Center on Aging.

[a] Division of General Internal Medicine, University of Utah School of Medicine, 5R218, Salt Lake City, UT 84132, USA; [b] Program in Molecular Medicine, University of Utah School of Medicine, 15 North 2030 East Rm 4145, Salt Lake City, UT 84112, USA
* Corresponding author. Department of Internal Medicine, Eccles Institute of Human Genetics, University of Utah, 15 North 2000 East, Suite 4220, Salt Lake City, UT 84112.
E-mail address: matthew.rondina@hsc.utah.edu

http://dx.doi.org/10.1016/j.mcna.2014.11.012
0025-7125/15/$ – see front matter © 2015 Elsevier Inc. All rights reserved.
medical.theclinics.com

of therapeutic agents available to providers. Nevertheless, the safe and effective use of NOACs in older adults remains less well established and understood, despite the marked increase in the prevalence of both AF and AF-associated thromboembolism (TE) in this population.[1–4] This review discusses strategies to assess bleeding and thrombosis risk in older adults with AF and summarizes pharmacologic options for the prevention of stroke, transient ischemic attack (TIA), and systemic embolism. The authors highlight practical considerations to the selection and use of these agents in older adults to aid clinical decision making.

MANAGEMENT GOALS

The aim of OAC is to prevent the devastating consequences of stroke in older adults with AF while minimizing complications from treatment. Older patients are at increased risk of bleeding complications, adding to the complexity of their treatment. The decision to use antithrombotic therapy in an individual patient with AF requires an estimate of the baseline stroke risk without treatment and the risk of bleeding (especially intracranial hemorrhage [ICH]) with treatment, followed by determination of the patient's values and preferences through shared decision making. Periodic reevaluation of the patient's stroke and bleeding risk is essential.[1] However, there are still important limitations to accomplishing these goals.

Stroke Risk Assessment

Stroke risk in individual patients with AF varies from less than 1% per year to more than 18% per year and depends on the presence, number, and relative predictive strength of different clinical risk factors for stroke and not on whether AF is paroxysmal, persistent, or permanent. The strongest risk factors are the presence of mechanical heart valves or mitral stenosis, and all patients with these require OAC.[1] For patients with nonvalvular atrial fibrillation (NVAF), the 4 strongest stroke predictors are prior stroke and/or TIA (relative risk [RR] = 2.5), hypertension (RR = 2.0), diabetes mellitus (RR = 1.7), and age (RR = 1.5 per decade).[2]

These clinical risk factors have been variably combined into different stroke risk stratification tools, including the $CHADS_2$ and CHA_2DS_2-VASc (**Tables 1** and **2**).[5,6] The CHA_2DS_2-VASc adds female sex, vascular disease, and age 65 to 74 years to the risk factors included in the $CHADS_2$ score. A systematic review of validation studies concluded that these 2 tools have the best, albeit modest, discrimination ability for stroke (c-statistics of 0.71 and 0.70, respectively).[7] Current clinical practice guidelines recommend the use of CHA_2DS_2-VASc over $CHADS_2$ because of several advantages.[1,8–10] Older age ($\geq$75 years) is the single most important risk factor for stroke (4.0%–5.0% per year; hazard ratio, 3.0–3.5), greater than hypertension, diabetes, or heart failure, thereby warranting extra weight (2 points) as a risk factor.[11,12] Although the 2 scores provide similar identification of patients with AF at high stroke risk, use of CHA_2DS_2-VASc improves stratification of patients considered low (score = 0) and intermediate (score = 1) risk by $CHADS_2$.[11,13] CHA_2DS_2-VASc identifies up to 22% of patients with AF with a $CHADS_2$ score of 0 whose annual event rate may not be low (0.84% for CHA_2DS_2-VASc score = 0 to 3.2% for CHA_2DS_2-VASc score = 3) and may benefit from OAC.[11,13] Thus, CHA_2DS_2-VASc better identifies the truly low risk cohort whose annual event rate is less than 1% and in whom anticoagulation can be safely deferred.[11,14,15]

Current guidelines for antithrombotic therapy in nonvalvular AF vary in their recommendations (**Table 3**).[1,8–10] For a CHA_2DS_2-VASc score of 0, no antithrombotic therapy (including no aspirin) is recommended. For a score of 2 or more, all recommend

Table 1	
CHADS$_2$ and CHA$_2$DS$_2$-VASc risk stratification score for stroke risk assessment in AF	
CHADS$_2$	
Risk Factor	**Score**
Congestive heart failure	1
Hypertension (>140/90)	1
Age ≥75 y	1
Diabetes mellitus	1
Stroke/transient ischemic attack/thromboembolism	2
Maximum Score	**6**
CHA$_2$DS$_2$-VASc	
Risk Factor	**Score**
Congestive heart failure	1
Hypertension	1
Age ≥75 y	2
Diabetes	1
Stroke/transient ischemic attack/thromboembolism	2
Vascular disease (prior myocardial infarction, peripheral arterial disease, or aortic plaque)	1
Age 65–74 y	1
Sex category (female sex)	1
Maximum Score	**9**

some form of OAC, with NOACs generally preferred over warfarin. However, there is no consensus on OAC for patients with a CHA$_2$DS$_2$-VASc score of 1. The 2014 American Heart Association/American College of Cardiology/Heart Rhythm Society guidelines suggest that clinicians consider the options of no antithrombotic therapy versus OAC versus aspirin for these patients.[1] In contrast, the 2014 National Institute for

Table 2			
Comparison of thromboembolic event rate by CHA$_2$DS$_2$-VASc score per 100 person years in 3 prospective real-world population cohorts			
CHA$_2$DS$_2$-VASc Score	**Friberg et al,[14] 2012**	**Singer et al,[15] 2013**	**Olesen et al,[11] 2011; 1-y Follow-up**
0	0.3	0.04	0.78
1	0.9	0.55	2.01
2	2.9	0.83	3.71
3	4.6	1.66	5.92
4	6.7	2.80	9.27
5	10.0	4.31	15.26
6	13.6	4.77	19.74
7	15.7	4.82	21.50
8	15.2	7.82	22.38
9	17.4	16.62	23.64

Data from Refs.[11,14,15]

Table 3
Antithrombotic therapy recommendations for nonvalvular atrial fibrillation

CHA_2DS_2-VASc Score	AHA/ACC/HRS 2014[1]	NICE 2014[8]	CCS 2012[8]	ESC 2012[7]
0	No Rx	No Rx	No Rx	No Rx
1	OAC or ASA or No Rx	Female sex: No Rx Male sex: Consider OAC	Age ≥65 y: NOAC preferred over VKA Vascular disease or female sex: ASA is a reasonable alternative	Female sex: No Rx Age ≥65 y or vascular disease: NOAC VKA with TTR >70% as an alternative to NOAC ASA only for patients who refuse or cannot tolerate OAC
≥2	OAC with warfarin, dabigatran, rivaroxaban, or apixaban	OAC with NOAC or VKA	OAC with NOAC preferred to VKA	OAC with NOAC VKA with TTR >70% as an alternative to NOAC

Abbreviations: ACC, American College of Cardiology; AHA, American Heart Association; ASA, aspirin; CCS, Canadian Cardiovascular Society; ESC, European Society of Cardiology; HRS, Heart Rhythm Society; Rx, treatment; NICE, National Institute for Health and Care Excellence; TTR, time in therapeutic range.
Data from Refs.[1,7,8]

Health and Care Excellence (NICE),[10] the 2012 Canadian Cardiovascular Society (CCS),[8] and the 2012 European Society of Cardiology (ESC)[9] guidelines recognize that women with AF younger than 65 years with no other stroke risk factors are at very low risk of stroke and should not receive any antithrombotic therapy.[16,17] The NICE guideline states that OAC be considered for men with a CHA_2DS_2-VASc score of 1, whereas the ESC recommends OAC for them. Because patients with AF aged 65 to 74 years with no other stroke risk factors have annual stroke rates of about 2% per year,[12] the CCS recommends OAC for them but not for patients whose only risk factor by CHA_2DS_2-VASc is female sex or vascular disease.

Bleeding Risk Assessment

The fatal or disabling bleeding risk of a patient with AF must be assessed when making decisions about antithrombotic therapy. A systematic review concluded that the HAS-BLED score (**Tables 4** and **5**) provides the best, although modest (c-statistic 0.58–0.80), estimation of major bleeding risk for warfarin OAC in patients with AF.[7,18] However, the HAS-BLED and other bleeding risk scores have important limitations. At least 80% of major bleeds predicted by these tools are extracranial hemorrhages (especially gastrointestinal [GI]) that carry low rates of mortality (<5%–6%) and rare disability.[19] Of much greater concern are ICHs, which constitute 15% to 20% of major bleeds during warfarin treatment and are responsible for 90% of fatal bleeds.[19] ICH carries rates of mortality and severe disability of 46% and 22%, respectively, in patients with AF treated with warfarin.[20]

None of the bleeding risk scores can quantitatively estimate absolute ICH risk nor can these scores identify patients with AF in whom the risk of ICH plus fatal or disabling extracranial hemorrhage is likely to exceed the risk of fatal or disabling ischemic stroke.

Table 4
The HAS-BLED bleeding risk score

Risk Factors	Score
Hypertension[a]	1
Abnormal liver[b] or kidney function[c]	1 or 2
Stroke	1
Bleeding[d]	1
Labile INR[e]	1
Elderly[f]	1
Drugs[g] or alcohol[h]	1 or 2

Abbreviation: INR, international normalized ratio.
[a] >160 mm Hg systolic.
[b] Cirrhosis, bilirubin >2 × ULN (upper limit of normal); aspartate aminotransferase/alanine aminotransferase/alkaline phosphatase >3 × ULN.
[c] Renal dialysis, history of renal transplant, or serum creatinine >2.26 mg/dL.
[d] Requiring hospitalization, decrease in hemoglobin >2 g/L, or requiring blood transfusion.
[e] Time in therapeutic range <60%.
[f] Age >65 years.
[g] Use of antiplatelet agents or nonsteroidal antiinflammatory drugs.
[h] >8 drinks per week.

In addition, these bleeding risk scores have been validated for warfarin OAC but not yet for NOACs. One recent guideline suggests that current bleeding risk scores do not have sufficient clinical utility to recommend their use.[1] Most current recommendations suggest that the HAS-BLED score not be used to exclude patients from OAC but rather to systematically identify and then eliminate modifiable bleeding risk factors such as uncontrolled hypertension, inadequate warfarin anticoagulation with labile international normalized ratios, unnecessary concomitant use of aspirin or nonsteroidal antiinflammatory drugs, and excessive alcohol use.[8–10]

PHARMACOLOGIC STRATEGIES

The elderly present a unique challenge in antithrombotic management because of the frequency of associated comorbidities that increase the risk of both stroke and bleeding, multiple drug therapy, concerns about compliance and cognitive impairment, low body weight, increased risk of falls, and decreased renal clearance of medications.

Oral Anticoagulation with Warfarin

Underutilization
Compared with no treatment, warfarin decreases the risk of stroke by approximately two-thirds and death by one-fourth, with an average number needed to treat (NNT) for 1 year to prevent 1 stroke of 37.[21] Despite compelling evidence of the benefits of warfarin on stroke prevention, it remains underutilized, with estimates that less than

Table 5
Major bleeding rates based on the HAS-BLED risk category

Score	Risk Category	Bleeds/100 Patient Years
0–1	Low	1.2–2.8
2	Moderate	3.6–5.4
≥3	High	6.0–9.5

half of eligible patients with AF without contraindications are receiving treatment.[22,23] The challenges with warfarin are well known and include unpredictable pharmacodynamics and pharmacokinetics, narrow therapeutic window, and numerous drug-drug and food-drug interactions, which necessitate frequent laboratory monitoring and dose adjustments.

Also contributing to suboptimal warfarin utilization are patient and physician fears of bleeding. Physicians are less likely to use anticoagulation in older patients, even in the absence of contraindications, because of the perception that the risks of treatment outweigh the benefits.[23,24] Each advancing decade of life is associated with a 14% reduction in warfarin use, independent of other risk factors for stroke.[3] In addition, patients frequently refuse anticoagulation. For example, one-third of patients enrolled in the apixaban versus acetylsalicylic acid to prevent stroke in atrial fibrillation patients who have failed or are unsuitable for vitamin K antagonist treatment (AVERROES) and atrial fibrillation clopidogrel trial with irbesartan for prevention of vascular events (ACTIVE A) studies refused a VKA because of the associated inconvenience and perceived bleeding risk.[25,26]

Fear of falls

Clinicians may disproportionately consider the risk of traumatic ICH from falls in their assessment of the net clinical benefit of OAC for older patients with AF. Clinician perception of fall risk is a key determinant in the decision to use OAC.[24] However, studies of patients with AF on OAC and who are at high fall risk do not consistently demonstrate an increased risk of traumatic ICH.[27] A modeling study suggested that patients with AF at a higher risk of stroke would have to fall greater than 295 times per year before the risk of traumatic ICH would exceed the risk of ischemic stroke; yet, in older persons who fall, the mean number of falls is only 1.8 per year.[28,29] In older Medicare beneficiaries with traumatic brain injury on OAC, resumption of warfarin therapy following hospital discharge resulted in a 17% reduction in the combined outcome of ischemic and hemorrhagic stroke.[30] Based on these data, many investigators propose that high fall risk is not a reason to avoid OAC.[10,27,28] For clinicians with significant concerns about individual patients, a referral to a faint and fall clinic or a comprehensive fall risk assessment can be considered.

Net clinical benefit of warfarin

Based on the need to balance the risks of ischemic TE with the risks of fatal and disabling major bleeding, prospective cohort studies of patients with AF have assessed the net clinical benefit of warfarin, which has been established as the annual rate of ischemic strokes prevented by warfarin minus the annual rate of ICH caused by warfarin, the latter multiplied by a factor of 1.5 to reflect the greater clinical severity of ICH than ischemic stroke.[16,31,32] Overall, the impact of warfarin is much higher on TE risk than on ICH risk.[31] Owing to increasing risk for stroke with aging and a constant increase in ICH risk with aging, the net clinical benefit of warfarin improves progressively with advancing age and is greatest for patients with AF 85 years and older.[31] Net clinical benefit of warfarin also improves progressively with major bleeding risk as measured by the HAS-BLED score; that is, warfarin OAC decreases ischemic stroke rate more than it increases ICH rate at all levels of bleeding risk.[16,32] Moreover, the net clinical benefit of warfarin is favorable in all groups except with CHA_2DS_2-VASc score of 0, confirming their truly low-risk status.[16,32] In this large study, only 0.4% of patients had a bleeding risk exceeding their stroke risk.[16] Thus, in almost all patients with AF, particularly the elderly and those at high bleeding risk, the risk of ischemic stroke without OAC exceeds the risk of intracranial bleeding with OAC.

Reflective of these data, the pendulum in antithrombotic management is swinging away from a focus on identifying high-risk patients for treatment with OAC and toward identification of the truly low-risk patient, in whom OAC can safely be deferred, while considering all other patients for anticoagulation treatment. Use of the CHA_2DS_2-VASc scoring system can help in identifying this subgroup of patients.

Antiplatelet Therapy

Aspirin monotherapy

In some settings, aspirin has been historically considered a safer alternative to OAC.[24] Aspirin was previously recommended for stroke prevention in patients considered low risk for stroke and seen as an acceptable alternative to OAC for patients at intermediate risk of stroke and for those who were deemed unsuitable for, or choose not to take, warfarin.[33] There is moderate evidence from numerous randomized controlled trials (RCTs) that aspirin decreases the risk of nonfatal stroke by 21% compared with no therapy but at a cost of a 50% to 60% increase in major extracranial bleeding.[21,34] However, in comparison to aspirin monotherapy, warfarin is superior, with a 37% greater reduction in strokes.[21] The RR of ICH is doubled with warfarin compared with aspirin, but this represents only a small absolute increase (0.2%–0.4% per year).[21]

Efficacy data for aspirin use in the elderly are even less compelling. In the Birmingham Atrial Fibrillation Treatment of the Aged (BAFTA) trial, patients aged 75 years or older were randomized to either warfarin or aspirin, 75 mg daily. Warfarin was associated with a significant reduction in fatal or disabling stroke, ICH, or systemic embolus (1.8% vs 3.8% per year; RR, 0.48; NNT, 50), with a similar risk of major hemorrhage.[35] The yearly risk of a major bleed on aspirin was not insignificant, at 2% per year.[35] Other studies have also demonstrated higher rates of side effects and intolerance to aspirin than warfarin.[36]

In a net clinical benefit analysis, aspirin was not found to be protective of TE, with an increased bleeding risk compared with no treatment, and a similar bleeding risk to warfarin, leading the investigators to suggest that aspirin should not be used for any patient with AF.[32] Aspirin is significantly less effective at stroke prevention than warfarin in older patients, with no difference in major bleeding.[4,35] In addition, the relative benefit of antiplatelet therapy has been shown to decrease significantly with age, but the relative benefit of warfarin does not.[4] Because stroke risk increases with age, the absolute benefit of OAC over antiplatelet therapy continues to increase as patients age.[4] Reflective of this, some guidelines no longer recommend use of aspirin as an acceptable alternative to OAC.[9,10,34]

Dual antiplatelet therapy

Compared with aspirin monotherapy, dual antiplatelet therapy offers superior stroke prevention (2.4% vs 3.3% per year; RR, 0.72), albeit as the expense of increased major bleeding (2.0% vs 1.3% per year; RR, 1.57) and ICH (0.4% vs 0.2% per year; RR, 1.87).[25] The atrial fibrillation clopidogrel trial with irbesartan for prevention of vascular events (ACTIVE W) trial evaluated dual antiplatelet therapy as a potential alternative to warfarin in patients with AF at high risk of stroke.[37] This trial was stopped early, as warfarin significantly reduced the risk of stroke by 42% compared with aspirin plus clopidogrel (3.93% vs 5.60% per year; NNT, 100), with no difference in mortality or major bleeding. Similar data were seen when apixaban was compared with the combination of aspirin and clopidogrel in the AVERROES trial, which was terminated prematurely because of a 50% reduction in stroke rate with apixaban, without any differences in bleeding. Apixaban was also associated with fewer adverse events and a lower rate of discontinuation.[26]

For patients who refuse OAC or are deemed unsuitable candidates for reasons other than bleeding risk, the combination of aspirin and clopidogrel should be considered, and this is now recommended in some guidelines over aspirin monotherapy.[9,34] Patients should be counseled that this regimen offers inferior stroke prevention compared with OAC, with no difference in bleeding risk.

Non-vitamin K–Dependent Oral Anticoagulants

The US Food and Drug Administration has approved 3 NOACs (dabigatran, rivaroxaban, and apixaban) for use in AF, with an additional agent (edoxaban) expected to be available in the near future (**Table 6**). These newer drugs provide clinicians with additional therapeutic options to prevent stroke in AF and lack many of the limitations inherent to warfarin. They have predictable pharmacodynamic and pharmacokinetic profiles, a wide therapeutic window, shorter half-life with rapid onset/offset of action, fewer drug-drug interactions, few to no food-drug interactions, no need for routine laboratory monitoring, and fixed dosing schedules.

Dabigatran is an oral direct thrombin inhibitor, whereas rivaroxaban, apixaban, and edoxaban are factor Xa inhibitors. Each of these drugs is either noninferior or superior to warfarin for stroke prevention, with markedly less intracranial bleeding (**Table 7**).[38–41] Dabigatran, rivaroxaban, and edoxaban caused higher rates of GI bleeding than warfarin. To better define the efficacy and safety of these medications in subgroups, meta-analyses of these phase 3 clinical trials have been performed.[42,43] NOACs are associated with an approximately 12% decrease in mortality compared with warfarin, a 20% decrease in stroke or systemic embolus, and, most impressively, a 50% reduction in ICH. The net clinical benefit of NOACs is not yet as clearly established as for warfarin. However, because of their 50% lower

Table 6
Comparison of NOACs for the prevention of stroke and systemic embolism in AF

	Rivaroxaban	Dabigatran	Edoxaban[b]	Apixaban
Prodrug or drug	Drug	Prodrug	Drug	Drug
Target	Factor Xa	Thrombin	Factor Xa	Factor Xa
Mean half-life (t $\frac{1}{2}$) (h)	7–11	12–17	9–11	8–15
Tmax (h)	2–4	0.5–2	1–2	3–4
Protein binding (%)	93	35	55	87
Dosing regimen[a]	20 mg daily	150 mg BID	Daily	5 mg BID
Dose adjustments	15 mg daily if CrCl 15–50	75 mg BID if CrCl 15–30	N/A	2.5 mg BID if ≥2 of the following: age ≥80 y, weight ≤60 kg, or serum creatinine ≥1.5 mg/dL
Major interactions	P-gp, CYP3A4	P-gp	P-gp	P-gp, CYP3A4
Estimated renal excretion (%)	66	80	35	25
Food effect	Delayed absorption	Delayed absorption	None	None

Abbreviations: BID, twice daily; CYP3A4, Cytochrome P450 3A4; P-gp, P -glycoprotein.
[a] US Food and Drug Administration–approved dosing.
[b] Edoxaban is not yet approved by US Food and Drug Administration, so no dose given.

Table 7
Summary of key, randomized clinical trials comparing NOACs to a VKA for the prevention of stroke and systemic embolism in AF

	Rivaroxaban	Dabigatran	Edoxaban	Apixaban
Phase 3 RCT	ROCKET AF	RE-LY	ENGAGE AF-TIMI 48	ARISTOTLE
Population	NVAF and $\geq$2 RF[a]	NVAF and $\geq$1 RF[a]	NVAF and CHADS$_2$ $\geq$2 RF	NVAF and $\geq$1 RF[a]
Patients, n	14,264	18,113	21,105	18,201
Study design	Double-blind, double-dummy	PROBE	Double-blind, double-dummy	Double-blind, double-dummy
Primary objective	Noninferior efficacy	Noninferior efficacy	Noninferior efficacy	Noninferior efficacy
Study drug dose(s)	20 mg daily	110 or 150 mg BID	60 mg daily	5 mg BID
Renal dose	15 mg daily	None	30 mg daily[b]	2.5 mg BID[c]
Age (y)	73.0	71.5	72.0	70.0
Male gender (%)	60.3	63.6	61.9	64.7
CHADS$_2$ score	3.5	2.1	2.8	2.1
TTR (%)	55	64	65	62
Aspirin use (%)	36.5	39.8	29.3	30.9

Abbreviations: ENGAGE AF-TIMI 48, effective anticoagulation with factor Xa next generation in atrial fibrillation–thrombolysis in myocardial infarction 48; NVAF, non-valvular atrial fibrillation; PROBE, prospective open-label blinded end point evaluation; RE-LY, randomized evaluation of long-term anticoagulation therapy.

[a] Risk factors (RF): age $\geq$75 y; history of stroke, transient ischemic attack, or systemic embolism; symptomatic heart failure and/or left-ventricular ejection fraction <40%; diabetes mellitus; and/or need for antihypertensive treatment.

[b] For patients with a CrCl 30–50 mL/min, a weight $\leq$60 kg, or the concomitant use of verapamil, quinidine, or dronedarone.

[c] For patients with two or more of the following criteria: an age of at least 80 years, a body weight of no more than 60 kg, or a serum creatinine level of 1.5 mg per deciliter (133 µmol per liter) or more.

risk of ICH, modeling analyses suggest that NOACs may provide even greater net clinical benefit than warfarin for patients with AF with a CHA$_2$DS$_2$-VASc score greater than or equal to 1.[44]

Efficacy and safety of non–vitamin K oral anticoagulants in older patients

Although there are no RCTs that have enrolled exclusively older patients with AF, the available evidence suggests that the safety and efficacy of NOACs in older adults is similar to the overall study population.[45] A meta-analysis of randomized trials of NOACs in patients 75 years or older showed significantly lower rates of stroke and systemic embolus than conventional treatment, with no increased risk of bleeding.[46] In the rivaroxaban once daily oral direct factor Xa inhibition compared with vitamin K antagonism for prevention of stroke and embolism trial in atrial fibrillation (ROCKET AF), the risk of any major bleeding was similar among patients who received rivaroxaban or warfarin, regardless of age, but intracranial bleeding was less with rivaroxaban.[39,47] In apixaban for reduction in stroke and other throm-boembolic events in atrial fibrillation (ARISTOTLE), the overall risk of stroke, death, and major bleeding increased with aging, but apixaban was more effective than warfarin in reducing these outcomes, irrespective of age.[40,48] Owing to increasing risk of stroke as patients age, the absolute benefit of NOACs over warfarin was greatest in the elderly. In contrast to rivaroxaban and apixaban, in the randomized evaluation of long-term anticoagulation therapy (RE-LY) trial, there was a highly significant interaction between treatment and age for major bleeding. In patients younger than 75 years, both doses of dabigatran were associated with a lower risk of major bleeding than warfarin. However, patients 75 years or older experienced similar rates of major extracranial bleeding compared with warfarin with dabigatran at a dose of 110 mg twice daily but a trend toward higher risk of extracranial bleeding with the dose of 150 mg twice daily. ICH was reduced with both doses of dabigatran compared with warfarin, regardless of age.[38,49] These data suggest that the safety of Xa inhibitors is less dependent on age than is dabigatran, with one possible explanation being that they are less dependent on renal clearance than dabigatran.[48]

Disadvantages of non–vitamin K oral anticoagulants

The potential disadvantages associated with the NOACs include twice daily dosing regimen (with the exception of rivaroxaban), short duration of action, lack of a reliable and readily available monitoring option, and lack of antidote (**Table 8**). Discussion of potential laboratory monitoring and reversal agents is beyond the scope of this article. The authors focus on renal impairment, because renal function declines with

Table 8
Considerations when choosing between a VKA and NOAC for older patients with AF

Consideration or Factor	Potentially Preferred OAC	Comment
Severe renal impairment (eg, CrCl 15–30 mL/min)	VKA, reduced-dose dabigatran 75 mg BID, or reduced dose rivaroxaban 15 mg daily	VKA elimination is independent of any renal impairment
End-stage kidney disease	VKA	VKA elimination is independent of any renal impairment
History of ICH	Dabigatran, rivaroxaban, apixaban, edoxaban	All NOACs reduced the risk of ICH compared with VKA
Mechanical heart valves	VKA	NOACs only approved in NVAF
Unstable INR or inability to comply with regular INR monitoring	Dabigatran, rivaroxaban, apixaban, edoxaban	Predictable Pharmacokinetics without need for routine monitoring
Poor adherence to taking medication	VKA	Longer half-life, ability to monitor compliance with INR
Concomitant use of azole antimycotics or ritonavir	Dabigatran, VKA	Azole antimycotics or ritonavir increase blood concentration of factor Xa inhibitors
Dyspepsia	VKA, rivaroxaban, apixaban, edoxaban	High incidence of dyspepsia with dabigatran
Poor compliance with twice daily medication	VKA, rivaroxaban	Once daily dosing regimen
History of GI bleeding	VKA, apixaban	Higher rates of GI bleeding with dabigatran, rivaroxaban, and edoxaban
Cost concerns	VKA	NOACs may be cost prohibitive to some patients

Abbreviations: CrCl, creatinine clearance; INR, international normalized ratio; NVAF, non-valvular atrial fibrillation.

advancing age and patients with severe renal impairment (creatinine clearance [CrCl] <30 mL/min, <25 mL/min for apixaban) were excluded from the clinical trials.

Non–vitamin K oral anticoagulants in older patients with renal impairment

NOACs have not yet been robustly studied in patients with severe renal impairment and are not recommended in patients with end-stage renal disease or undergoing hemodialysis. The incidence of renal impairment increases with age, and renal impairment increases the risk of both TE and bleeding complications in patients with AF independent of other risk factors.[49,50] Because AF is primarily a disease of the elderly, these two conditions often coexist, leading to significant concerns about bleeding risk. In the RE-LY trial, patients on either dabigatran or warfarin with a CrCl less than 50 mL/min experienced a 2-fold higher risk of major bleeding compared with those who had a CrCl of 80 mL/min or more.[49] In the ROCKET AF trial, reduced-dose rivaroxaban in patients with CrCl 30 to 49 mL/min preserved the benefit over warfarin without increasing bleeding and with fewer fatal bleeds.[51] In ARISTOTLE, apixaban reduced the rate of stroke, death, and major bleeding compared with warfarin regardless of renal function, including in patients older than 75 years.[48,50] Thus, all 3 trials showed higher rates of bleeding and stroke with impaired renal function regardless of randomized treatment assignment, suggesting no increased risk with NOACs as compared with warfarin.

Although NOACs seem to be at least as safe as warfarin in the short term and reduce the risk of intracranial bleeding, longer-term data are still needed. There may also be subtle differences between the NOACs in rates of ischemic stroke, myocardial infarction, bleeding, and death, but the lack of head-to-head trials makes this difficult to discern. Nevertheless, when considered overall, the significant decrease in ICH, fixed dosing schedules, lack of routine laboratory monitoring, and fewer drug-drug interactions make the NOACs an attractive alternative to warfarin for some older patients (see **Table 8**).

FUTURE CONSIDERATIONS AND SUMMARY

In summary, age remains one of the strongest risk factors for stroke in patients with AF. The use of guideline-recommended stroke scoring systems, in combination with a bleeding risk factor assessment, can help guide providers in determining the net clinical benefit of antithrombotic therapy in older adults with AF. Recently approved NOACs may offer select advantages for the prevention of stroke and systemic embolism in older patients with AF. Future studies may further elucidate the net clinical benefit of NOACs in the elderly and help guide more individualized AC selection and management.

ACKNOWLEDGMENTS

We thank Dr Barry Stults for his valuable comments and expert suggestions.

REFERENCES

1. January CT, Wann LS, Alpert JS, et al. 2014 AHA/ACC/HRS guideline for the management of patients with atrial fibrillation: a report of the American College of Cardiology/American Heart Association Task Force on practice guidelines and the Heart Rhythm Society. J Am Coll Cardiol 2014;64(21):2246–80.
2. Stroke Risk in Atrial Fibrillation Working Group. Independent predictors of stroke in patients with atrial fibrillation: a systematic review. Neurology 2007;69(6):546–54.
3. Brophy MT, Snyder KE, Gaehde S, et al. Anticoagulant use for atrial fibrillation in the elderly. J Am Geriatr Soc 2004;52(7):1151–6.

4. van Walraven C, Hart RG, Connolly S, et al. Effect of age on stroke prevention therapy in patients with atrial fibrillation: the atrial fibrillation investigators. Stroke 2009;40(4):1410–6.
5. Gage BF, Waterman AD, Shannon W, et al. Validation of clinical classification schemes for predicting stroke: results from the National Registry of Atrial Fibrillation. JAMA 2001;285(22):2864–70.
6. Lip GY, Nieuwlaat R, Pisters R, et al. Refining clinical risk stratification for predicting stroke and thromboembolism in atrial fibrillation using a novel risk factor-based approach: the Euro Heart Survey on atrial fibrillation. Chest 2010;137(2): 263–72.
7. Lopes RD, Crowley MJ, Shah BR, et al. Stroke prevention in atrial fibrillation. Rockville (MD): Agency for Healthcare Research and Quality (US); 2013.
8. Skanes AC, Healey JS, Cairns JA, et al. Focused 2012 update of the Canadian Cardiovascular Society atrial fibrillation guidelines: recommendations for stroke prevention and rate/rhythm control. Can J Cardiol 2012;28(2):125–36.
9. Camm AJ, Lip GY, De Caterina R, et al. 2012 focused update of the ESC Guidelines for the management of atrial fibrillation: an update of the 2010 ESC Guidelines for the management of atrial fibrillation. Developed with the special contribution of the European Heart Rhythm Association. Eur Heart J 2012;33(21):2719–47.
10. Jones C, Pollit V, Fitzmaurice D, et al. The management of atrial fibrillation: summary of updated NICE guidance. BMJ 2014;348:g3655.
11. Olesen JB, Lip GY, Hansen ML, et al. Validation of risk stratification schemes for predicting stroke and thromboembolism in patients with atrial fibrillation: nationwide cohort study. BMJ 2011;342:d124.
12. Olesen JB, Fauchier L, Lane DA, et al. Risk factors for stroke and thromboembolism in relation to age among patients with atrial fibrillation: the Loire Valley Atrial Fibrillation Project. Chest 2012;141(1):147–53.
13. Olesen JB, Torp-Pedersen C, Hansen ML, et al. The value of the CHA2DS2-VASc score for refining stroke risk stratification in patients with atrial fibrillation with a CHADS2 score 0-1: a nationwide cohort study. Thromb Haemost 2012;107(6): 1172–9.
14. Friberg L, Rosenqvist M, Lip GY. Evaluation of risk stratification schemes for ischaemic stroke and bleeding in 182 678 patients with atrial fibrillation: the Swedish Atrial Fibrillation cohort study. Eur Heart J 2012;33(12):1500–10.
15. Singer DE, Chang Y, Borowsky LH, et al. A new risk scheme to predict ischemic stroke and other thromboembolism in atrial fibrillation: the ATRIA study stroke risk score. J Am Heart Assoc 2013;2(3):e000250.
16. Friberg L, Rosenqvist M, Lip GY. Net clinical benefit of warfarin in patients with atrial fibrillation: a report from the Swedish Atrial Fibrillation cohort study. Circulation 2012;125(19):2298–307.
17. Avgil Tsadok M, Jackevicius CA, Rahme E, et al. Sex differences in stroke risk among older patients with recently diagnosed atrial fibrillation. JAMA 2012; 307(18):1952–8.
18. Pisters R, Lane DA, Nieuwlaat R, et al. A novel user-friendly score (HAS-BLED) to assess 1-year risk of major bleeding in patients with atrial fibrillation: the Euro Heart Survey. Chest 2010;138(5):1093–100.
19. Fang MC, Go AS, Chang Y, et al. Death and disability from warfarin-associated intracranial and extracranial hemorrhages. Am J Med 2007;120(8):700–5.
20. Fang MC, Go AS, Chang Y, et al. Thirty-day mortality after ischemic stroke and intracranial hemorrhage in patients with atrial fibrillation on and off anticoagulants. Stroke 2012;43(7):1795–9.

21. Hart RG, Pearce LA, Aguilar MI. Meta-analysis: antithrombotic therapy to prevent stroke in patients who have nonvalvular atrial fibrillation. Ann Intern Med 2007; 146(12):857–67.
22. Ogilvie IM, Newton N, Welner SA, et al. Underuse of oral anticoagulants in atrial fibrillation: a systematic review. Am J Med 2010;123(7):638–45.e4.
23. Waldo AL, Becker RC, Tapson VF, et al. Hospitalized patients with atrial fibrillation and a high risk of stroke are not being provided with adequate anticoagulation. J Am Coll Cardiol 2005;46(9):1729–36.
24. Pugh D, Pugh J, Mead GE. Attitudes of physicians regarding anticoagulation for atrial fibrillation: a systematic review. Age Ageing 2011;40(6):675–83.
25. Investigators A, Connolly SJ, Pogue J, et al. Effect of clopidogrel added to aspirin in patients with atrial fibrillation. N Engl J Med 2009;360(20):2066–78.
26. Connolly SJ, Eikelboom J, Joyner C, et al. Apixaban in patients with atrial fibrillation. N Engl J Med 2011;364(9):806–17.
27. Donze J, Clair C, Hug B, et al. Risk of falls and major bleeds in patients on oral anticoagulation therapy. Am J Med 2012;125(8):773–8.
28. Man-Son-Hing M, Nichol G, Lau A, et al. Choosing antithrombotic therapy for elderly patients with atrial fibrillation who are at risk for falls. Arch Intern Med 1999;159(7):677–85.
29. Tinetti ME, Speechley M, Ginter SF. Risk factors for falls among elderly persons living in the community. N Engl J Med 1988;319(26):1701–7.
30. Albrecht JS, Liu X, Baumgarten M, et al. Benefits and risks of anticoagulation resumption following traumatic brain injury. JAMA Intern Med 2014;174(8): 1244–51.
31. Singer DE, Chang Y, Fang MC, et al. The net clinical benefit of warfarin anticoagulation in atrial fibrillation. Ann Intern Med 2009;151(5):297–305.
32. Olesen JB, Lip GY, Lindhardsen J, et al. Risks of thromboembolism and bleeding with thromboprophylaxis in patients with atrial fibrillation: a net clinical benefit analysis using a 'real world' nationwide cohort study. Thromb Haemost 2011; 106(4):739–49.
33. Singer DE, Albers GW, Dalen JE, et al. Antithrombotic therapy in atrial fibrillation: American College of Chest Physicians Evidence-Based Clinical Practice Guidelines (8th Edition). Chest 2008;133(Suppl 6):546S–92S.
34. You JJ, Singer DE, Howard PA, et al. Antithrombotic therapy for atrial fibrillation: antithrombotic therapy and prevention of thrombosis, 9th ed: American College of Chest Physicians evidence-based clinical practice guidelines. Chest 2012; 141(Suppl 2):e531S–75S.
35. Mant J, Hobbs FD, Fletcher K, et al. Warfarin versus aspirin for stroke prevention in an elderly community population with atrial fibrillation (the Birmingham Atrial Fibrillation Treatment of the Aged Study, BAFTA): a randomised controlled trial. Lancet 2007;370(9586):493–503.
36. Rash A, Downes T, Portner R, et al. A randomised controlled trial of warfarin versus aspirin for stroke prevention in octogenarians with atrial fibrillation (WASPO). Age Ageing 2007;36(2):151–6.
37. ACTIVE Writing Group of the ACTIVE Investigators, Connolly S, Pogue J, et al. Clopidogrel plus aspirin versus oral anticoagulation for atrial fibrillation in the Atrial fibrillation Clopidogrel Trial with Irbesartan for prevention of Vascular Events (ACTIVE W): a randomised controlled trial. Lancet 2006;367(9526): 1903–12.
38. Connolly SJ, Ezekowitz MD, Yusuf S, et al. Dabigatran versus warfarin in patients with atrial fibrillation. N Engl J Med 2009;361(12):1139–51.

39. Patel MR, Mahaffey KW, Garg J, et al. Rivaroxaban versus warfarin in nonvalvular atrial fibrillation. N Engl J Med 2011;365(10):883–91.
40. Granger CB, Alexander JH, McMurray JJ, et al. Apixaban versus warfarin in patients with atrial fibrillation. N Engl J Med 2011;365(11):981–92.
41. Giugliano RP, Ruff CT, Braunwald E, et al. Edoxaban versus warfarin in patients with atrial fibrillation. N Engl J Med 2013;369(22):2093–104.
42. Dentali F, Riva N, Crowther M, et al. Efficacy and safety of the novel oral anticoagulants in atrial fibrillation: a systematic review and meta-analysis of the literature. Circulation 2012;126(20):2381–91.
43. Miller CS, Grandi SM, Shimony A, et al. Meta-analysis of efficacy and safety of new oral anticoagulants (dabigatran, rivaroxaban, apixaban) versus warfarin in patients with atrial fibrillation. Am J Cardiol 2012;110(3):453–60.
44. Banerjee A, Lane DA, Torp-Pedersen C, et al. Net clinical benefit of new oral anticoagulants (dabigatran, rivaroxaban, apixaban) versus no treatment in a 'real world' atrial fibrillation population: a modelling analysis based on a nationwide cohort study. Thromb Haemost 2012;107(3):584–9.
45. Deedwania PC. New oral anticoagulants in elderly patients with atrial fibrillation. Am J Med 2013;126(4):289–96.
46. Sardar P, Chatterjee S, Chaudhari S, et al. New oral anticoagulants in elderly adults: evidence from a meta-analysis of randomized trials. J Am Geriatr Soc 2014;62(5):857–64.
47. Goodman SG, Wojdyla DM, Piccini JP, et al. Factors associated with major bleeding events: insights from the ROCKET AF trial (rivaroxaban once-daily oral direct factor Xa inhibition compared with vitamin K antagonism for prevention of stroke and embolism trial in atrial fibrillation). J Am Coll Cardiol 2014;63(9):891–900.
48. Halvorsen S, Atar D, Yang H, et al. Efficacy and safety of apixaban compared with warfarin according to age for stroke prevention in atrial fibrillation: observations from the ARISTOTLE trial. Eur Heart J 2014;35(28):1864–72.
49. Eikelboom JW, Wallentin L, Connolly SJ, et al. Risk of bleeding with 2 doses of dabigatran compared with warfarin in older and younger patients with atrial fibrillation: an analysis of the randomized evaluation of long-term anticoagulant therapy (RE-LY) trial. Circulation 2011;123(21):2363–72.
50. Hohnloser SH, Hijazi Z, Thomas L, et al. Efficacy of apixaban when compared with warfarin in relation to renal function in patients with atrial fibrillation: insights from the ARISTOTLE trial. Eur Heart J 2012;33(22):2821–30.
51. Fox KA, Piccini JP, Wojdyla D, et al. Prevention of stroke and systemic embolism with rivaroxaban compared with warfarin in patients with non-valvular atrial fibrillation and moderate renal impairment. Eur Heart J 2011;32(19):2387–94.

Sleep Problems in the Elderly

Juan Carlos Rodriguez, MD[a,b,c,]*, Joseph M. Dzierzewski, PhD[a,b],
Cathy A. Alessi, MD[a,b]

KEYWORDS

• Sleep problems • Sleep apnea • Insomnia • Older adults • Diagnosis and treatment

KEY POINTS

• Older adults frequently have sleep problems, such as sleep apnea and insomnia. These problems are often unrecognized and undertreated.
• Obstructive sleep apnea (OSA) has been associated with hypertension, coronary artery disease, depression, car accidents, cognitive impairment, stroke, and mortality.
• Positive airway pressure therapy effectively treats OSA.
• Insomnia carries many negative unwanted consequences in older adults. Psychological techniques have been shown to be effective and should be considered as the first-line therapy for older adults with insomnia.

INTRODUCTION

Sleep problems are not an inherent part of the aging process.[1,2] Many older adults have good sleep quality until the end of their lives. It is critical that sleep problems are not mistaken for physiologic changes in sleep-awake patterns and sleep architecture that occur throughout the lifespan.[3,4] Older adults often display an advanced circadian tendency, having an earlier bedtime and an earlier wake-up time. Sleep architecture changes include spending an increased proportion of time in stages N1 and N2 sleep (ie, the lighter stages of sleep), a decreased proportion of time in stage N3

This work was supported by UCLA Claude D. Pepper Older Americans Independence Center (NIA 5P30 AG028748); NIH/NCATS UCLA CTSI (UL1TR000124); the VA Advanced Geriatrics Fellowship Program; the Geriatric Research, Education, and Clinical Center (GRECC); and the VA Greater Los Angeles Healthcare System.
a Geriatric Research, Education, and Clinical Center, VA Greater Los Angeles Healthcare System, 16111 Plummer Street (IE), North Hills, Los Angeles, CA, USA; b Department of Medicine, David Geffen School of Medicine, University of California, Los Angeles, 405 Hilgard Avenue, CA 90095, USA; c Department of Medicine, Pontificia Universidad Catolica de: Ave, Libertador Bernardo O'Higgins 340, Santiago, Chile
* Corresponding author. VA Greater Los Angeles Healthcare System, 16111 Plummer Street (11E), North Hills, CA 91343.
E-mail address: juan.rodrigueztapia@va.gov

sleep (ie, a deeper stage of sleep) and in rapid eye movement (REM) sleep. These architecture changes reflect a decrease in deep, restorative sleep and an increase in light, transitory sleep. In addition, older adults tend to spend slightly less time asleep than their younger counterparts. Although some older adults complain of poor nighttime sleep or subsequent impairments in daytime functioning, others assume that their difficulties are part of the normal aging process. Therefore, a focused evaluation of sleep, specifically sleep apnea and insomnia, and related daytime functioning should be performed in every older adult in whom sleep disturbances are suspected.

SLEEP APNEA

Patients with sleep apnea show repetitive episodes of reduction (hypopnea) or absence (apnea) of airflow during sleep. There are 2 main types of sleep apnea: obstructive and central sleep apnea. In obstructive sleep apnea (OSA), the upper airway is obstructed secondary to anatomic factors, such as obesity and/or reduced activation of the dilatory muscles of the airway (eg, under the effect of alcohol or sedative drugs). In OSA, the respiratory effort persists during the episodes of hypoventilation. In contrast, central sleep apnea (CSA) is secondary to a reduced respiratory effort secondary to problems such as neurologic conditions (eg, stroke) or heart failure. Other causes of CSA include drugs or substances that depress the central nervous system (eg, opioids). Adverse effects associated with sleep apnea include hypertension, coronary artery disease, depression, car accidents, cognitive impairment, stroke, and mortality.

Diagnosis

Common symptoms of sleep apnea are daytime sleepiness, irritability, fatigue, and headache. Frail older patients may report subtle manifestations or may even be asymptomatic. Common findings at the physical examination include a crowded oral pharynx, obesity, and hypertension. However, obesity is less common in elderly patients with OSA. It is important to interview bed partners, because they can describe snoring, apnea episodes, or irritability. Sleep apnea can easily be screened for using clinical prediction rules such as the STOP-BANG questionnaire (**Box 1**).[5] However, the

---

Box 1
STOP-BANG questionnaire

1. Do you snore loudly (loud enough to be heard through closed doors, or for your bed partner to elbow you for snoring at night)?

2. Do you often feel tired, fatigued, or sleepy during the daytime (such as falling asleep while driving)?

3. Has anyone observed you stop breathing or choke/gasp during your sleep?

4. Are you or are have you been treated for high blood pressure?

5. Body mass index more than 35 kg/m^2?

6. Age older than 50 year old?

7. Neck size (measure around Adams apple) larger than 43 cm (17 inches) for men or 41 cm (16 inches) for women?

8. Male gender?

Fewer than 3 "Yes" answers indicates low risk for sleep apnea.
Courtesy of www.stopbang.ca; with permission.

gold standard for the diagnosis of sleep apnea is in-laboratory polysomnography. This test provides information regarding sleep stages, muscular activity, nasal airflow, oxygen saturation, electrocardiogram, snoring, body position, and limb movements.[6] Portable monitors used at home are a simpler and more economical alternative. The concordance rates between home sleep tests and polysomnography are high, especially for moderate and severe cases of sleep apnea.

Sleep Apnea Severity

Sleep apnea is classified into severity levels based on the average number of hypopneas and apneas per hour during sleep (apnea hypopnea index [AHI]) as either mild (AHI 5–15), moderate (AHI 16–30), or severe (AHI>30).

Treatment

Positive airway pressure (PAP) is the first-line therapy for patients with moderate or severe sleep apnea. PAP maintains the airway open during sleep through administration of air pressure. Some of the benefits observed with the use of PAP are improvement of sleep quality, daytime symptoms, blood pressure, ventricular ejection fraction, and cognitive function. Moreover, PAP decreases the risk of stroke, cardiovascular disease, and mortality in older patients.[7,8] Continuous PAP (CPAP) is the most commonly used type of PAP. CPAP provides a fixed pressure of air during the breathing cycle. There are more advanced devices (eg, biphasic PAP or auto adjusting positive airway pressure [APAP]) that can provide different levels of pressure and may be better tolerated by some patients. Good adherence (ie, >4 hours of use per night on 70% of nights) to PAP prescription may be a challenge to older patients. Long-term adherence is best predicted by the use of PAP during the first week. There are several features of PAP machines that may improve patient compliance, such as humidifiers, ramp, and pressure relief. In addition, there are several mask options and sizes available to better fit patient preferences (eg, nasal or facial mask). In addition, concomitant psychological cognitive behavior therapy may improve adherence. For patients with obstructive apnea who reject or do not adhere to PAP therapy, oral appliances (ie, mandibular advancement devices) may be an alternative. These devices move the jaw forward in the hope of reducing airway obstruction. Other treatment alternatives (eg, nose valves and uvulopalatopharyngoplasty surgery) have not been extensively evaluated in older adults. General recommendations for older patients with sleep apnea, including those with mild sleep apnea, are avoidance of sedative drugs and alcohol, reducing weight, and controlling blood pressure.

INSOMNIA

According to the International Classification of Sleep Disorders, Third Edition,[9] insomnia is defined as a subjective complaint of difficulty initiating sleep, difficulty maintaining sleep, or early morning awakenings that occur at a minimum of 3 nights per week, for 3 months, and are associated with significant daytime consequences. Examples of these daytime consequences include difficulty concentrating, mood disturbances, fatigue, and worry about sleep. On average, older adults experience insomnia symptoms for several years before receiving a formal diagnosis.[10] Insomnia often occurs in association with other clinical disorders (eg, comorbid insomnia) especially in older people. Insomnia prevalence tends to be higher in older individuals with multiple physical and psychiatric conditions (60% or more), and higher among older women than among older men.[3,11] The higher prevalence of insomnia among older adults is thought to be a consequence of the physical and mental health comorbidities of aging, rather than a consequence of aging itself.[12] Negative consequences of insomnia in late life include decreased quality of life, risk for falls, psychological and physical difficulties, economic and social costs, risk for nursing home placement, and mortality.

Diagnosis

An examination of sleep quality should be performed during routine clinical visits in older patients. Asking about sleep satisfaction and sleep-related daytime consequences may alert the provider to the necessity of a more a structured clinical interview focusing on insomnia symptoms. The clinical interview for insomnia should focus on probable predisposing factors, precipitating factors, and perpetuating factors (ie, the 3 P model, **Fig. 1**).[13] Predisposing factors include risk factors that increase older adults' likelihood of experiencing poor sleep, such as poor physical and mental health, family history of insomnia, or low socioeconomic status. Precipitating factors include any events that can acutely disrupt sleep, such as recent life events (eg, depressive episode, hospitalization, loss of a loved one, moving residences). Perpetuating factors are the aspects of the older adult's daily behavior that serve to maintain poor sleep, and include all contextual, emotional, and behavioral influences.

Some self-report questionnaires, such as the Insomnia Severity Index[14] (**Box 2**), have been validated in older adults. However, the retrospective recall of sleep quality necessary for these questionnaires may be difficult for older adults. A daily sleep diary can capture useful information regarding sleep timing, quantity, and quality across consecutive days. The use of a daily sleep diary is recommended in the clinical diagnosis of insomnia in late life. Polysomnography and wrist actigraphy are not indicated for the diagnosis of insomnia in older adults.

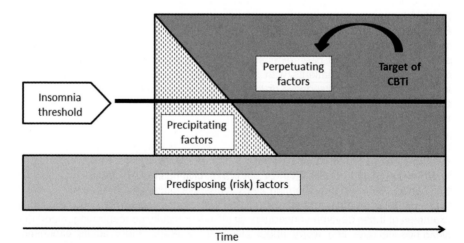

Fig. 1. The 3 P conceptual model of insomnia. Predisposing factors: physical and mental health, family history of insomnia, poverty, and so forth. Precipitating factors: depressive episode, hospitalization, loss of a loved one, moving, and so forth. Perpetuating factors: spending too much time in bed, not following a regular sleep schedule, and so forth. CBTi, Cognitive behavior treatment of insomnia.

Box 2
Insomnia Severity Index

Please rate the current (ie, last 2 weeks) severity of your insomnia problems:

1. Have you had difficulty falling asleep?

2. Have you had difficulty staying asleep?

3. Have you had problems waking up too early?

4. How satisfied/dissatisfied are you with your sleep pattern?

5. How noticeable to others do you think your sleep problem is in terms of impairing the quality of your life?

6. How worried/distressed are you about your current sleep problem?

7. To what extent do you consider your sleep problem to interfere with your daily functioning (eg, daytime fatigue, mood, ability to function at work/daily chores, concentration, memory)?

Five-point Likert scale (0, no problem; 4, very severe problem) possible answers for all items. Total score categories: 0 to 7, no clinically significant insomnia; 8 to 14, subthreshold insomnia; 15 to 21, moderate insomnia; 22 to 28, severe insomnia.
Courtesy of Charles M. Morin, PhD, Quebec QC; with permission.

Treatment

Insomnia should be treated with a specific and focused plan. Treatment of late-life insomnia can involve psychological strategies, pharmacologic agents, or both. In general, psychological techniques should be considered as initial treatment methods because of their strong empirical evidence, high safety in older adults, and long-term benefits. Psychological treatment approaches have outperformed pharmacologic treatment in head-to-head trials, and are also better than combined psychological/pharmacologic therapy.[15,16]

Psychological interventions

Psychological interventions for insomnia encompass a variety of different techniques, including sleep education, cognitive therapy, sleep hygiene, relaxation strategies, stimulus control, sleep restriction, and multicomponent treatment packages (eg, cognitive behavior treatment of insomnia [CBTi]). Sleep is largely behaviorally regulated, with a strong homeostatic biological drive and circadian component. Interventions with a foundation in behavioral theory and practice have been proved to be effective in the management of insomnia.

Stimulus control is a behavioral strategy based on classic conditioning principles that is intended to increase the response of sleep associated with the stimulus of the bed and bedroom. There is strong evidence in support of stimulus control for insomnia in late life.[17,18] Sleep restriction is a behavioral strategy designed to increase the homeostatic sleep drive and strengthen the circadian signal through more closely aligning time spent in bed with time spent asleep. There is strong evidence in support of sleep restriction for insomnia in late life.[17,18] Sleep education, cognitive therapy, and sleep hygiene have little empirical evidence to support their use as stand-alone treatment options for insomnia in older adults. These three techniques are most useful in combination with other psychological treatment strategies. Note that, although sleep hygiene recommendations are the most commonly used nonpharmacologic treatment approach to the management of insomnia, there is no evidence to support the use of sleep hygiene alone for insomnia management. Sleep hygiene recommendations are commonly used as the control or placebo condition in psychological intervention research. Relaxation strategies may prove beneficial alone in improving the sleep of older adults. However, like the strategies mentioned earlier, relaxation techniques may be most useful in combination with other psychological treatments.

CBTi has the strongest empirical grounding of all available behavioral treatment options for insomnia in older adults.[17,18] CBTi is a combination treatment of insomnia typically consisting of stimulus control and sleep restriction, and variations of CBTi also include psychoeducation and cognitive therapy. CBTi has been shown to result in large improvements in perceived sleep in older adults with insomnia, and older adults prefer CBTi to sedative hypnotics. The typical delivery of CBTi involves one-on-one, face-to-face delivery in 4 to 6 weekly (or biweekly) sessions each lasting between 30 and 60 minutes. CBTi has been successfully delivered in as little as one or two 30-minute sessions, in group formats, and over virtual communication lines. Although commonly delivered by specially trained clinical psychologists, CBTi has been successfully administered by supervised nurse practitioners, health educators, and older adult peers. The overwhelming confluence of evidence supports CBTi as the recommended treatment of insomnia in older adults. **Table 1** provides a comprehensive listing of psychological treatment options for insomnia in late life.

Pharmacotherapy

Medication treatment of late-life insomnia should be used in the minority of patients; however, sedative hypnotic medications are the most commonly prescribed treatment approach for insomnia in older patients. Older adults are more than twice as likely as younger adults to be prescribed medication treatment of insomnia,[19] which is particularly concerning given the increased risk for drug side effects, drug interactions, tolerance and dependence, and lack of empirical evidence supporting long-term use in older patients. In general, short-term pharmacotherapy may be indicated in situations of acute insomnia. In older adults with chronic insomnia, sedative hypnotics should be used with great caution. When the decision is made to prescribe a sedative hypnotic to an older patient, the smallest effective dose with the lowest risk of adverse effects should be prescribed for the shortest duration of time.

The commonly used sedative hypnotic medications can be broadly grouped into 3 categories: (1) short, intermediate, and long-acting benzodiazepines; (2) nonbenzodiazepines or z-drugs; and (3) sedating antidepressants. In general, long-acting benzodiazepines should not be used with older adults because of increased risks of daytime sedation, falls, and confusion. Short-acting or intermediate-acting benzodiazepines are preferable for patients with a primary complaint of sleep maintenance difficulties. The nonbenzodiazepines have a shorter duration of action than the benzodiazepines and are thought to carry a lower side effect profile; however, there is a limited amount of evidence pertaining directly to the use of most nonbenzodiazepines specifically in older patients with comorbid insomnia. Sedating antidepressants (eg, trazodone, tricyclics) are often used off-label for their sedative hypnotic effects, although little empirical evidence supports the use of sedating antidepressants as hypnotic agents in older adults. In addition, agents with anticholinergic side effects should be avoided (eg, diphenhydramine).

Differential Diagnosis of Sleep Apnea and Insomnia

Differential diagnosis for sleep apnea and insomnia includes distinguishing these two common sleep disorders from other sleep disturbances in late life. Less common sleep disorders in older adults include:

- Circadian rhythm sleep disorders: older people commonly experience an advanced sleep phase (ie, an early bedtime and early morning awakening). Sleep

Table 1
Psychological treatment approaches for insomnia in older adults

Technique	Level of Support
Sleep education Information regarding normal sleep changes with age. Designed to normalize current sleep, improve expectations, and reduce anxiety	Low[a]; not an evidence-based practice[b]; not a recommendation[c]
Cognitive therapy Maladaptive thoughts, beliefs, and attitudes can negatively affect sleep. Challenging these thoughts can help promote sleep through a reduction in sleep disruptive thoughts and emotions	Low[a]; not an evidence-based practice[b]; not a recommendation[c]
Sleep hygiene Instruction to avoid or limit sleep disruptive substances and behaviors, including caffeine, alcohol, nicotine, exercising, and heavy meals at night	Low[a]; not an evidence-based practice[b]; not a recommendation[c]
Relaxation strategies Active or passive relaxation techniques all designed to reduce physiologic or mental arousal that may be interfering with sleep	Moderate[a]; not an evidence-based practice[b]; standard recommendation[c]
Stimulus control Behavioral technique based on classic conditioning principals. Instructs individuals to limit their use of the bed to sleep and sex, and to limit the amount of time spent awake in bed	Strong[a]; not an evidence-based practice[b]; standard recommendation[c]
Sleep restriction Behavioral strategy designed to match the amount of time spent in bed with the amount of time asleep. A consistent sleep schedule and time in bed is collaboratively prescribed and adjusted as needed	Strong[a]; evidence-based practice[b]; guideline recommendation[c]
Multicomponent treatment packages Combines several individual components into a treatment package. Usually consists of stimulus control and sleep restriction. Sometimes includes sleep education, cognitive therapy, relaxation techniques, or sleep hygiene recommendations	Strong[a]; evidence-based practice[b]; standard recommendation[c]

[a] Based on the authors' critical review of empirical evidence and clinical practice with older adults.
[b] Criteria for an intervention to be considered evidence-based include 50% of the outcome measures showing significant treatment effects with between-group effect sizes of at least 0.20.[17]
[c] American Academy of Sleep Medicine practice parameters.[18]

logs can be used for making a diagnosis and for monitoring treatment response. Wrist actigraphy or polysomnography is indicated when the diagnosis is unclear or another sleep disorder is suspected.

- REM behavior disorder (RBD): patients act out dreams with forceful movements and behaviors during sleep secondary to a lack of the normal muscle atonia present during REM sleep. They may injure themselves or their bed partners. RBD is rare in the general population, but has been associated with dementia, multiple system atrophy, and Parkinson disease. Polysomnography is required to confirm the diagnosis and to rule out other conditions.

- Restless legs syndrome (RLS): RLS is an uncontrollable urge to move the legs, commonly caused by an uncomfortable sensation in the legs. The symptoms start during periods of rest (especially at night) and are partially or entirely relieved with movement. RLS is diagnosed clinically based on symptoms.

SUMMARY/FUTURE CONSIDERATIONS

Sleep problems are frequent, but underexplored in older adults. Sleep apnea and insomnia are particularly important sleep problems in older adults. Both sleep apnea and insomnia are associated with serious negative physical, mental, and social consequences. Methods for recognition of these disorders are effective, and safe treatment options are available. Improving the adherence to PAP therapy and reducing the use of sedative drugs are important goals to address in clinical practice and future research with older adults.

REFERENCES

1. Foley DJ, Monjan AA, Brown SL, et al. Sleep complaints among elderly persons - an epidemiological study of 3 communities. Sleep 1995;18:425–32.
2. Mellinger GD, Balter MB, Uhlenhuth EH. Insomnia and its treatment: prevalence and correlates. Arch Gen Psychiatry 1985;42:225–32.
3. Morgan K. Sleep and aging. In: Lichstein K, Morin C, editors. Treatment of late-life insomnia. Thousand Oaks (CA): Sage Publications; 2000. p. 3–36.
4. Floyd JA, Medler SM, Ager JW, et al. Age-related changes in initiation and maintenance of sleep: A meta-analysis. Res Nurs Health 2000;23:106–17.
5. Chung F, Yegneswaran B, Liao P, et al. STOP Questionnaire: a tool to screen for obstructive sleep apnea. Anesthesiology 2008;108:812–21.
6. Epstein LJ, Kristo D, Strollo PJ Jr, et al. Clinical guidelines for the evaluation, management and long-term care of obstructive sleep apnea in adults. J Clin Sleep Med 2009;15:263–76.
7. Campos-Rodriguez F, Pena-Grinan N, Reyes-Nuñez N, et al. Mortality in obstructive sleep apnea-hypopnea patients treated with positive airway pressure. Chest 2005;128:624–33.
8. Giles TL, Lasserson TJ, Smith BJ, et al. Continuous positive airway pressure for obstructive sleep apnoea in adults. Cochrane Database Syst Rev 2006;(25):CD001106.
9. Diagnostic Classification Steering Committee TMJC. International classification of sleep disorders. 3rd edition. Rochester (NY): American Academy of Sleep Medicine; 2014.
10. Dzierzewski JM, O'Brien E, Kay DB, et al. Tackling sleeplessness: psychological treatment options for insomnia in older adults. Nat Sci Sleep 2010;2:47–61.
11. Ford DE, Kamerow DB. Epidemiological study of the sleep disturbances and psychiatric disorders. JAMA 1989;262:1479–84.
12. Vitiello MV, Moe KE, Prinz PN. Sleep complaints cosegregate with illness in older adults: clinical research informed by and informing epidemiological studies of sleep. J Psychosom Res 2002;53:555–9.
13. Spielman AJ, Caruso LS, Glovinsky PB. A behavioral perspective on insomnia treatment. Psychiatr Clin North Am 1987;10:541–53.
14. Bastien CH, Vallieres A, Morin CM. Validation of the Insomnia Severity Index as an outcome measure for insomnia research. Sleep Med 2001;2:297–307.

15. Morin CM, Colecchi C, Stone J, et al. Behavioral and pharmacological therapies for late life insomnia: a randomized controlled trial. JAMA 1999;281:991–9.
16. Sivertsen B, Omvik S, Pallesen S, et al. Cognitive behavioral therapy vs zopiclone for treatment of chronic primary insomnia in older adults. JAMA 2006;295:2851–8.
17. McCurry SM, Logsdon RG, Teri L, et al. Evidence-based psychological treatments for insomnia in older adults. Psychol Aging 2007;22:18–27.
18. Morgenthaler T, Kramer M, Alessi CA, et al. Practice parameters for the psychological and behavioral treatment of insomnia: an update. An American Academy of Sleep Medicine report. Sleep 2006;29:1415–9.
19. Stewart R, Besset A, Bebbington P, et al. Insomnia comorbidity and impact and hypnotic use by age group in a national survey population aged 16 to 74 years. Sleep 2006;29:1391–7.

Index

Note: Page numbers of article titles are in **boldface** type.

Med Clin N Am 99 (2015) 441–450
http://dx.doi.org/10.1016/S0025-7125(15)00012-7
0025-7125/15/$ – see front matter © 2015 Elsevier Inc. All rights reserved.

Moving?

Make sure your subscription moves with you!

To notify us of your new address, find your **Clinics Account Number** (located on your mailing label above your name), and contact customer service at:

Email: journalscustomerservice-usa@elsevier.com

800-654-2452 (subscribers in the U.S. & Canada)
314-447-8871 (subscribers outside of the U.S. & Canada)

Fax number: 314-447-8029

Elsevier Health Sciences Division
Subscription Customer Service
3251 Riverport Lane
Maryland Heights, MO 63043